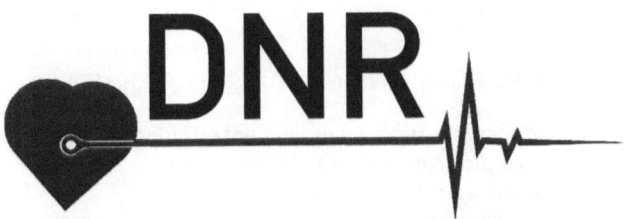

DNR

DO NOT RESUSCITATE

A novel by

Geraldine M. McEachern

DNR: Do Not Resuscitate, published April, 2024
Editorial and proofreading services: Kathleen A. Tracy, Cath Lauria , Katie Barger
Interior layout and cover design: Howard Johnson
Front cover artwork: designed by Freepik.com
Interior artwork (title page and chapter openers): designed by Freepik.com
Photo Credits: Author photo owned by Geraldine M. McEachern

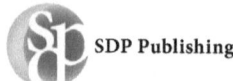 **SDP Publishing**

Published by SDP Publishing, an imprint of SDP Publishing Solutions, LLC.

ISBN-13 (print): 979-8-9885439-1-6

ISBN-13 (ebook): 979-8-9885439-2-3

Library of Congress Control Number: 2024901894

Printed in the United States of America

For Brian McEachern and Marie C. Duffield who had the fortitude and presence to transition to DNR before they lost the ability to do so.

Acknowledgments

I would like to acknowledge all the nurses I worked with (during the '70s and '80s), especially my mentors Marie C. Duffield RN and Gail A. Woodhead RN They were the epitome of passionate caregivers and taught me how to prioritize my nursing skills to care for the sickest patients in the Coronary Intensive Care Unit and to observe for the unapparent. Physician colleagues too numerous to mention worked very long hours beside us and still managed to teach the medical staff and patients in a very caring, compassionate way.

Also to former Mayor Raymond L. Flynn, who was always a staunch supporter of nurses.

I would like to thank Lisa Akoury-Ross and her team of editors for guiding me through the arduous process of refining my manuscript for publication. Lisa patiently walked me through the process and answered my endless questions. I am very grateful for their insight and expertise.

To the patients and their families, I deeply respect and appreciate that they allowed us to care for them when many of the scientific developments in medicine were in the neophyte stages of extending their life expectancy.

For those patients who were not DNR and had no voice but remained in a vegetative state, I hope freedom came with your last breath.

A Word from the Author

To be human is to be mortal. Despite that knowledge, people manage to go about their daily lives without obsessing over their inevitable demise. If we were to dwell on dying, not only would we miss out on making the most of the time we do have, but we'd probably be miserable and neurotic. So we tuck that knowledge away and keep it at arm's length as long as we possibly can.

What we don't imagine is something many people would consider worse than death: being brought back to "life" through modern techniques of resuscitation despite part or all of the brain suffering catastrophic damage after an unexpected, violent snap of fate's fingers.

Unless a patient has a *Do Not Resuscitate* medical bracelet on when they come through hospital emergency room doors, they will be resuscitated if they code. On the one hand, who has the right to deny anyone, regardless of how long he has been without a heartbeat, a chance to come back through resuscitative efforts? On the other hand, is existing in an essentially vegetative or uncommunicative state really being alive? It is a legal, moral, and ethical quandary.

DNR, set in the mid 1970s and '80s, will take you on a journey into the realm between what we call life and what we pronounce as death. While fictional, it is based on a truth that any of us could one day face.

Prologue

She was 87 years old with sparkling blue eyes. Her pale complexion was softened by her wavy salt and pepper hair. There was a calmness about her that bespoke wisdom. Heart monitors were measuring her rhythm after sustaining a heart attack. Not long after arriving in the Coronary Care Unit her heart rate suddenly slowed to a flatline. CPR was immediately initiated. Her left hand remained clenched to the bedside rail with the sun radiating off her gold wedding band. After a few minutes of CPR her heart rate came back, and she woke up and looked around at the medical team and smiled.

The nurse manager whispered in her ear, "Where were you?" She stated, "I was flying over Castle Island near where I live." After that episode, the attending cardiologist sat on the edge of her bed and spoke with her. She declared herself a DNR and died peacefully three days later with her son at her side.

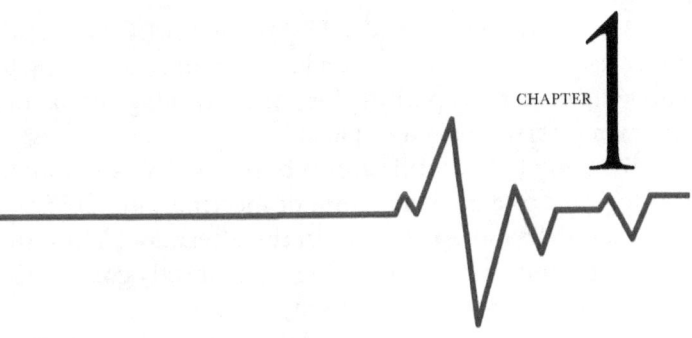

CHAPTER 1

John

The day began with my usual routine. My faithful alarm clock woke me at 6:30 a.m. Although morning is not for everyone, I relished the few moments of solitude offered by the early hours. Once my feet were firmly on the floor I took a cold shower to get my blood pumping, followed by a hearty breakfast with my family where we discussed our itinerary.

It was a Wednesday morning like any other. My wife, Linda, and I were teasing one another about how long it had been since we'd been out to dinner without the children. We made spontaneous plans to have my mom look after the kids and meet for dinner, just the two of us, at a new Mexican restaurant in Harvard Square that evening. In keeping with my morning caffeine ritual, I drove off to work, drinking my second cup of coffee along the way.

I felt extremely happy. Spring was approaching, and the trees and shrubs along the Charles River were sprouting their first greenery of the season. The warmer, longer days had tulips inching their way above the earth. It felt good to be alive.

As commissioner of the Department of City Health Services, I was able to bypass a long line of cars waiting to enter the enormous parking lot—the advantage of having my own reserved parking space.

Entering the administrative building, I was not looking forward to a busy morning of meetings, lunch at city hall, and then more meetings in the afternoon. Thinking of that glorious sunshine outside, I reluctantly got into the elevator that would take me to my office.

I watched the floor numbers light up until the elevator came to a quiet halt on the fifth floor. Walking down the narrow corridor to my office, I began to notice a dull ache in my jaw. It had come and gone over the last few days, especially when I was feeling stressed or racing from one meeting to the next. It felt like a toothache and I treated it as such, making an appointment with the dentist for later that week. I never mentioned it to anyone else since I didn't think it was a big deal; it never persisted for an extended period of time.

However, today was different. While I was sipping my third cup of coffee, the pain came and went repeatedly. Toward the end of the day, it had increased in such frequency that it was almost beyond bearable.

Cutting my last meeting short, I finally called one of the doctors in the dental clinic room to see if there was a dentist on duty. I was told that one of the oral surgeons would be coming by in an hour, and I could be seen then. An hour sounded like forever to me, so I took a couple of aspirins and got cleaned up to meet Linda for dinner.

To my relief after a few minutes of rest, the pain subsided on its own. That convinced me it was nothing more than a toothache relieved by aspirin and rest, so there was no need for a trip to the emergency room. I went to my car and headed for the expressway.

Listening to the distressing news events of the day on the radio, I made my way onto the ramp to the expressway.

Traffic was unusually heavy, and I wished I had driven across town rather than fighting my way through it. I made very little headway, and with each passing minute my tension increased because I knew there was no way I would be on time for dinner.

I was so stressed I even considered leaving my car in the breakdown lane, walking back down the up ramp, and taking the train. Knowing this was an absurd idea and that I probably wouldn't have a car when I returned, I simply sat and waited. And waited.

The car inched its way forward, going nowhere fast. Some people can calmly wait through traffic until it subsides, and others get all worked up over it. I was always in the latter group. What made it even worse was not wanting Linda to wait a long time for me to show up, and a long time it was going to be. The fumes from the close proximity of the cars began to get to me, and I found myself becoming uncontrollably agitated.

The pain in my jaw abruptly returned, only this time it was accompanied by a stab of pain in the left side of my chest that just wouldn't quit. It felt as though someone was standing on my chest. The pain was awful. I had never experienced anything like it. I managed to tolerate it for the first few minutes, but it soon got so bad I couldn't drive anymore.

I somehow managed to steer the car into the breakdown lane, continually repeating: *I can make it. I can make it.*

Safely out of traffic I rested my head on the steering wheel, hoping it would ease the pain. Perspiration dripped from my brow, and I thought I was going to pass out. I was terribly nauseous and thought if only I could vomit, the pain would go away.

A young man passing by in a black van stopped and asked me if I was okay. After describing to him what I was experiencing, he told me to stay put and that he would call 911 for an ambulance. I did not discourage it. I knew something was dreadfully wrong.

I wanted to vomit so badly. I remember opening the car door to put my feet out and get as much air as I could because it was becoming difficult to breathe. Then like a shot there was an explosion of lights, the deafening sound of sirens, the outcry of voices—and total darkness.

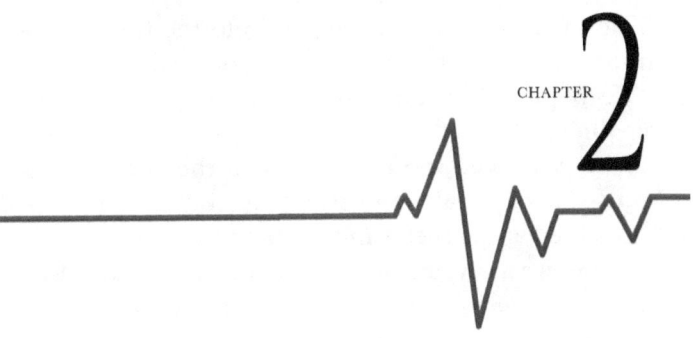

ICU

Reporters were already gathering on the sidewalk closest to the emergency entrance. Someone had leaked to the press that the commissioner had suffered a heart attack on the expressway and was in an ambulance on his way to the hospital.

Just moments earlier the paramedics had called in on the red phone, which is connected to all City Health Service ambulances, to alert the trauma room that a critical case was incoming so the emergency room personnel could prepare. Soon the succinct, high pitch of the ambulance siren could be heard approaching.

Flashing red lights bathed the patient receiving area as the ambulance cautiously backed up to the doors where doctors and nurses stood waiting. When the ambulance came to a halt, the driver raced out of his seat to open the back doors. Inside, the second EMT was performing chest compressions on the unconscious commissioner, whose pale face was covered with blood and vomit.

The medical team rushed him into the trauma area, with the attending physician barking out orders.

"Keep pumping, keep pumping, and get him into Room One fast!"

As they walked the EMT updated the doctor on the commissioner's vitals and what treatments they had administered at the scene and along the way.

"When we arrived on the expressway, he was still conscious and suffering from severe chest pain. He arrested on us just as we were getting him from the car onto the stretcher, so we intubated him and established an airway."

The chief resident nodded and told one of the nurses, Marsha, to prepare a syringe of epinephrine to inject directly into the commissioner's heart. Then he turned to one of the residents.

"Jake, get off the rest of his clothes. What's his rhythm now?"

"He's still flatlined."

"Get that neckline in. Did someone call for a respirator?"

"Yes, Doctor."

The attending injected the epinephrine, then the nurse administered the remaining drugs.

"Okay, stop pumping for a second," the attending said, looking at the monitor. "It looks as though he has something. Okay, let's shock him; give him the full blast. Everybody back."

They applied the paddles to the commissioner's chest and released a four-hundred-watt jolt, causing the commissioner's body to jerk stiffly into the air. The electrocardiograph indicated an irregular rhythm.

"Give him a milligram of atropine," the attending said. After the dose was administered, he asked, "Does he have blood pressure and a pulse with this, Jake?"

"I feel a weak femoral pulse, but he has no blood pressure that I can hear."

They watched and waited, then saw the commissioner's heartbeat suddenly speed up to 160 beats a minute.

"I can hear the blood pressure now," Jake announced. "It's about seventy over fifty."

"Good. Let's put him on low-dose dopamine to see if we can raise the blood pressure a bit," the attending said, his shoulders finally relaxing. But as he looked around the room for the Coronary Care Unit resident, his body tensed again. "Where the hell is the CCU resident? He should have been down here by now."

"He just called a few moments ago and said he was on his way," Marsha said. "Apparently, they had an emergency up there just before all this happened."

"Okay. Did the paramedic take a cardiogram before the patient flatlined.?"

Marsha nodded. "I believe I saw it on top of the desk."

"Would you get it for me?"

"Sure."

A moment later the CCU resident ran up. The attending turned to him with crossed arms. "Well, hello, Mac. I am glad you finally arrived."

"Sorry for the delay, David, but we have one guy who keeps going in and out of v-tach."

"That's okay. Take a look at this. It's truly an impressive cardiogram."

"Jesus! He has an anterior wall infarction."

"Yeah, it was tough getting him back. He was flatlined for a while." The attending pointed to the commissioner's legs, which looked still, with his feet pointed downward. "He's having some decerebrate posturing."

"That is not a good sign. Why don't we get a CAT scan of his brain before we move him to the CCU? Just in case. He's the commissioner and should have everything done."

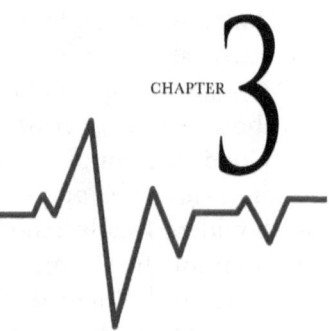

CHAPTER 3

John

As I was being lifted into the ambulance, the flashing red lights faded further and further away from me. I lapsed into a peacefulness I had never experienced before. It wasn't frightening, and in fact I fought not to return. But just as I was approaching a warm, glowing light, I was jolted away from the experience.

My mind seemed awake and alert, but I had no control over my body. I could hear voices all around, but I could not speak. My only thoughts were: *Why are they doing this to me? Why are they bringing me back?*

Then the voices stopped. I had no idea of time. It could have been minutes, hours, or days before I heard the same voices begin again. I still couldn't move.

"Mr. West? Mr. West, can you hear me? Squeeze my finger if you can hear me and understand."

I tried, oh God, did I try. But my fingers wouldn't work.

"Does he respond, Marsha?"

"No, Mac, there's nothing yet."

I was completely motionless. I was so scared. What the hell was happening to me? I knew I must be in some type of coma. *Why am I not waking up? Why could I hear and not speak? Why? Why me?* I wondered what the hell life was supposed to be now.

I wanted to cry but couldn't do that either. There I was, half man, half dead. Why didn't they let me die? I felt myself begin to drift into a heavy sleep, as though drugged, traveling back in time through my dreams to when I was a teenager living with my parents at the old homestead.

Our house was nestled on a narrow road densely lined by huge maples that intertwined with one another forty feet in the air during summertime. Our seven-room bucolic, vintage colonial New England home had a massive chimney that soared out of the roof toward the sky.

Mom's garden friends would always remark about the eye-catching, brightly polished, brass pineapple door knocker affixed to the solid wood front door. She explained that it was an old custom and meant that our house was one of gracious hospitality.

As long as I lived there, Mom and Dad never turned anyone away who was in need. Even though Dad was a doctor with a very busy schedule, if anyone came to our door for help, he would immediately stop what he was doing to give aid.

We lived on a well-tended acre of land surrounded by a three-foot white picket fence. I loved the gate to that fence, which let me wander as I pleased. Mom was not too crazy about the easy accessibility I had, never knowing when I would slip out to visit Mary Ellen Brougham, who lived down the street. We had grown up together and became the best of friends. We were virtually inseparable and did everything together, sharing a special camaraderie.

However, as teenagers our feelings transformed into a yearning for one another. Mary Ellen had a delicate, creamy complexion, striking long strawberry blond hair, and an insatiable desire to be an actress.

I had my dad's thick, black, curly hair, his good looks, and his tall, broad-shouldered physique, reaching almost six feet by the time I was fifteen. I considered myself very lucky; my younger brother, Sam, was short and chubby with a big nose. Nobody could figure out where he'd acquired that nose.

Even though I was becoming a young man, Mom still didn't want me out too late after dark. I kept testing her anyway until I'd hear her melodious voice calling my name. Then it was time to get home.

"Got to go, Mary Ellen. Mom is calling me."

"Will I see you tomorrow, Johnny?"

"You bet, right after breakfast."

I remember the night when I told my mom I thought I was in love with Mary Ellen. I'd run home as fast as I could and found Mom waiting patiently at the front door.

"Johnny, you know better than to stay out this late after dark."

"But, Mom, I was just down the street at Mary Ellen's."

"I don't care. You have responsibilities. Why, you haven't even touched your homework."

"Okay, Mom, you win."

I went upstairs and tried to concentrate on my studies but couldn't. I quietly tiptoed back downstairs and poured myself a glass of milk.

"Johnny, you have not been upstairs five minutes with your homework. What on earth is the matter with you?"

"Mom, I think I'm in love."

"In love?" She laughed lyrically.

"Mom, I'm serious. Mary Ellen is the most beautiful girl I know."

"She's only fourteen years old, and you're just fifteen."

"Soon to be sixteen," I protested, feeling defensive.

"I'm old enough to know what I feel. And I want to be with her every moment I can. And she feels the same."

"Never you mind, Johnny West. Just behave with that girl. Now go upstairs and focus on your homework."

Late that evening, it began to snow lightly. My dad still wasn't home, but that was nothing new. His devotion to his patients meant he often stayed at work late, tending to their more urgent needs. However, he would usually phone if he was going to be extraordinarily delayed.

The phone rang at ten-thirty. Within seconds, I heard Mom cry from downstairs.

"Johnny! Get your coat and hurry."

Her tone scared me, and I almost fell down the stairs in my haste. "Mom, what is it?"

In a trembling voice, she said, "Your dad was just taken to Woodville Hospital. They think he might have had a heart attack."

She roused my ten-year-old brother Sam our of a sound sleep and rushed him over to our next-door neighbor, Mrs. Wright. Then we sped to the hospital. We drove in silence, our sense of dread palpable. I prayed as we sped along the snow-covered streets.

My God, please don't take him. I need him so much.

When we arrived at the hospital, Mom asked that I wait for her outside the ladies' room before going to see him. When she came out, she looked like a new woman. She'd dried her tears and applied some makeup and was ready to take this straight on for Dad's sake.

We checked in at the front desk to find out where Dad was and, with trepidation, headed for his room. He was lying quietly with an oxygen mask on. His face was a pale gray color, and his lips seemed to quiver.

Mom laid her head on his chest and put her arms around his shoulders as if to cradle him. She whispered softly to him. "Lance, honey, I love you. You'll pull through this and be just fine."

As she kissed him on the forehead, the tears she tried so hard to control started rolling down her face. "Johnny is here too."

I moved to his bedside. He motioned for my hand. We locked fingers and tears slid from his eyes. I felt more of a man that day than ever before.

"I love you, Dad."

He looked at me and smiled. I knew he understood.

Dad made a miraculous recovery and came home three weeks after his heart attack, the day before his fifty-sixth birthday. He literally walked on eggshells for the next four weeks until he began to gain some strength and courage.

He was eventually able to go back to work at his practice, but his doctors had warned him that he had to cut back. So instead of his usual 24/7 workaholic schedule, he now worked just four hours a day. He was not happy about it but would begrudgingly growl that it was better than nothing.

Mom assumed more responsibilities, including becoming Dad's personal secretary. They appeared to enjoy each other more than they used to. After so many years of him never being home, they finally had time—richly deserved—to spend with one another. At times it seemed as though they were like teenagers in love again, renewing themselves within each other.

My sixteenth birthday arrived none too soon. Mom, Dad, and Sam planned a birthday party for me, inviting a few aunts, uncles, and of course, Mary Ellen. It was a small celebration but a big day in my life. I was now eligible for my learner's permit, and two months later I obtained my driver's license.

Full of exuberance and confidence, I took Mary Ellen for a long Sunday drive upcountry. It was the middle of spring, with everything bursting with life around us. Small fluffy white clouds danced in the bright blue sky.

We found a little lake near the mountains that was so peaceful and serene it seemed covered in glass.

We dashed out of the car and spread our picnic out on the green grass. Mary Ellen, with the help of her mother, had packed chicken, potato salad, pickles, and homemade apple pie.

As we ate, I asked, "Mary Ellen, do you think my father would have let me take the car so soon if he didn't think I was responsible?"

"He knows you are bright, dependable, and growing into a fine young man."

"Do you think of me as a young man?"

"In more ways than one, Johnny West."

"Really?"

"You've grown so much and taken over plenty of responsibility since your father took ill. Come on, let's go for a swim."

The first plunge into the lake was so cool and refreshing. We were able to swim to a small waterfall pouring out from the rocks and forest above. I didn't realize what was happening at first, but when we swam back to the tiny beach bordering the lake, I was looking at Mary Ellen not as a high school sweetheart but as a woman.

Her body was so streamlined in her bathing suit, with just enough of her soft milky white breasts to intrigue me. Oh, how I wanted to be with her. I quickly let the thought pass; she was still fifteen.

We dried ourselves and went for a walk in the woods. She talked and talked as we ambled along about her aspirations of becoming an actress. When Mary Ellen saw my amused expression, she got annoyed.

"You watch, Johnny. Someday, I'll be a famous actress."

"I have no doubt. I'm just teasing you. If there's one person in this world you'll have complete support from, it's me."

We continued our walk silently, arm in arm, occasionally taking the time to gaze at the countryside instead of each other. It was six o'clock when we arrived back home that evening. I longed for the day that I could take Mary Ellen into my arms and make love to her.

The following morning at breakfast I asked Mom for sone advice about college, knowing full well her choice, as well as my own, was Harvard.

"Mom, what do you think of me applying to Harvard after high school? I know it's Dad's alma mater, and I think he would be honored."

"Johnny, I don't think anything would please us more. Your father would be very proud of you. Do you have any other choices in mind?"

"Notre Dame, but I'm going to try my best to enter Harvard."

"With the cost of education today and your dad hardly working, you'll have to apply for a scholarship or grant to match the funds your father and I can give you."

"Don't worry, Mom. I'll fill out the applications and try my best."

Try my best I did. The library was full of names and places that awarded scholarships for college. I must have mailed out fifteen applications. After many days of anxiously awaiting the mailman, I finally received an acceptance. To Harvard University.

The Harvard Alumni Fund, established in the latter part of the 1800s, awarded me a $6,000 scholarship to be applied toward the first two years of tuition. Beyond belief, my father matched the same amount for the following two years and added a little extra spending money. I was on cloud nine, even more so because Notre Dame had accepted me as well.

The months passed, and the day I had waited so long for finally came—I entered Harvard. I was assigned a roommate in the dormitory. His name was Bill Hadley from Dorchester. Students had the option of asking for a new roommate if they weren't a good match, but Bill and I took to one another from the start. We both enjoyed the classes we were taking and the social life. I also had a part-time job on the weekends at a drug store in Harvard Square.

At the end of the first semester I came home for Christmas vacation. Thanks to my job I was able to buy some Christmas presents. In the short time I'd been away, Dad had grown visibly older and weaker. He was shuffling from room to room whereas before he would sprint. I didn't understand what was happening to him.

While Dad was taking an afternoon nap, I finally summoned the nerve to ask my mom.

She gently took me by the hand into my room and then explained that his heart was failing. She told me they had seen specialists, but there was nothing they could do for him.

I couldn't believe it; he had seemed so strong before I left for college.

"He can only do so much now," Mom continued. "He needs all the support he can get from us."

I started to cry, and Mom comforted me as always.

Christmas Day arrived. We exchanged gifts and sat down for a huge turkey dinner. Dad barely ate, though, and when dinner was over he shuffled to his rocking chair, which is where he spent most of his time.

I would go kneel beside him, and sometimes we reminisced about old times. He'd often fall asleep, but I would continue talking. I think he enjoyed that.

Mary Ellen came over on New Year's Eve so we could ring in the new year together. Dad had gone upstairs to watch Guy Lombardo's celebration on TV in their bedroom while I regaled Mom and Mary Ellen with stories about my first semester in college, including my initiation into one of the Harvard fraternities, which was somewhat of an embarrassing ordeal.

"I could not enter the fraternity if I did not come back with six one-dollar bills, and believe me, they were watching all the time. It was early morning, the day after Halloween, and pouring rain like the devil. I approached six business-men for a dollar each, all the while explaining to them that it was a contribution for me to go to Clown School. They either felt sorry for me or thought I was crazy, I never knew which, but thank God they all gave me a dollar."

Mary Ellen could not stop laughing, which was con-tagious.

"Johnny, I can't believe they made you do that."

"Well, I'll tell you, that was mild compared to some of the things they made others do."

About fifteen minutes before the stroke of midnight, Mom poured herself and Dad a glass of their favorite brandy and headed upstairs, discretely leaving Mary Ellen and me alone.

But when she walked into the bedroom, she found that Dad had died peacefully in his sleep. I guess we were somewhat prepared—as prepared as anyone is to accept the finality of death.

Mary Ellen was by my side through that trying time. Mom spent many hours alone in her room. My younger brother Sam had a difficult time and didn't stop crying for days. We grew closer as a family than we ever had before.

When I announced that I wouldn't be returning to Harvard so that I could help her and Sam, my mom shouted, "Absolutely not! Your father worked too hard for you to throw your college education away."

After she calmed down, she apologized for raising her voice at me and then explained that even through grief and loss, life must continue.

During the entire second semester, I had not seen Mary Ellen. I came home that following summer with one year at Harvard under my belt and began to work for a small construction company for the summer.

On the second day after my return I surprised Mary Ellen with my arrival. I was walking toward her house when a figure silhouetted against the sun came toward me and bounded into my arms. I picked her up, and we kissed and hugged for so long that we forgot we were out in the middle of the street. Her mother was out on the porch calling for us to come in.

"Welcome home, Johnny. Have some lemonade," she said. "How is school?"

"Coming along pretty well, Mrs. Brougham. It feels so good to be home for the summer."

Mary Ellen's mother was a nice woman, a devout Irish Catholic who loved to cook and do her work around the house and garden. We enjoyed the lemonade on that hot day and sat for hours talking about our experiences at school. It was a memorable afternoon.

Mary Ellen and I left her mother's house at dusk and went for a walk, talking over old times and new. We were growing into adults and were still crazy in love.

That summer our vacation took us to the cottage my paternal grandfather had built. It was on Cape Cod in Harwich Port, which burst alive with energy in the summertime after the long New England winter's nap. Summer cottages are passed down from generation to generation, and the atmosphere is one of friendliness, warmth, and good old down-home hospitality.

Mom used to own a small boutique in the center of town when she and Dad were first married. Even though it was only open in the summertime, when they decided to have children Mom felt her first responsibility was to us, so she sold the shop. But she would sigh every time we walked past the building.

Our cottage was situated right on the beach, surrounded by high sand dunes.

Mary Ellen came down that summer around the middle of July. I took two weeks off from my summer construction job to spend with her. I was so eager to get there and see Mary Ellen. While driving I started daydreaming about having my arms around her and almost had an accident. One thing I did not like about the Cape was the constant flow of stop-and-go traffic in summer.

Everyone was in good spirits, enjoying the bright sunshine and warm breezes. That afternoon we all went sailing. With Dad no longer with us, I was now the skipper of the boat. With full sails up and approaching the open ocean, Mom seemed engulfed by the sea. By her expression you could see that she longed for Dad to be with us. When she caught me staring at her, she broke her reverie.

"Well, children, what are your plans for the future?" she asked Mary Ellen and me.

Before anyone had a chance to answer, Sam blurted out: "I'm going to be a doctor, Mom. A brain surgeon."

"Really? Why are you choosing that?"

"I just want to help people."

"I'm sure you will, Sam."

From the time he was in first grade, Sam was always good with his hands. His fingers were extremely nimble, enabling him to perform precise movements. Dad would always let him help adjust the office equipment. Handling it with the utmost care, he would be done in no time at all. Not me, though. I was always fumbling to get the right nut and bolt in place.

"What about you, Johnny? What are your plans?" Mom asked.

"I don't know exactly yet. I do know I would like to finish Harvard and get my business degree. After that, I'm not sure."

"By then, I'm sure you will know, honey. It's wise to take your time now and think it through."

"I'm going to be an actress, Mrs. West."

"Truly, Mary Ellen?"

"Yes. I've been in a couple of school plays and have

done well. When I enter college this fall, drama will be my major subject."

"That'll be hard work, Mary Ellen, along with all your other studies."

"I know, but I feel I can do it."

"Well, I hope all your dreams come true for all of you. My prayers will be with you always."

We returned that evening feeling an inner peace within ourselves, especially Mom, whose beautiful glow was back on her face. After we secured the boat and were on our way back to the cottage, I asked Mary Ellen if she'd like to go for a walk.

"You don't think it is getting too dark, do you?"

"No, of course not. The only thing to fear is the night sharks."

"That's not funny, Johnny West."

We walked through the narrow pathway that led to the now moonlit beach, arm in arm. I broke the silence.

"Have you ever fantasized about making love?"

Mary Ellen looked up at me. "Sometimes, especially when I lay awake in bed in the dark and think of how I wish things were."

"I can't think of anything else lately than to have my arms around you."

"Oh, Johnny, I feel the same way."

The only sound was the ocean's rolling surf. We sat down on the dunes under a beautiful night sky, the stars pulsing as if communicating with one another. A warm breeze caused the dune grass to rustle behind us. I turned to look at Mary Ellen's moonlit face and put my arms around her. My lips met hers, and we lowered ourselves onto the sand.

A rush of heat warmed my body. When I whispered my desire to make love, Mary Ellen responded by unbuttoning my shirt. Nervously and tenderly, we undressed one another, then kissed and embraced one another naked in the sand. We took it slowly, savoring each sensation. I caressed and kissed her breasts, which were even more beautiful than I had imagined. She took me into her hand, and I felt myself grow harder with each gentle stroke.

"Oh, God, Mary Ellen ... this is so beautiful."

Our lips only parted for me to kiss her breasts and rest my face in her neck. I rolled on top of her, rocking slowly, my erection stimulating her over and over. Our breathing got heavier, and our hearts pounded rapidly with arousal. Mary Ellen's rhythmic breathing turned into a loud moan as I entered her.

It was finally happening. We moved as one, reached orgasm as one, and became one. After a moment I rolled onto my back, the sand cool against my hot skin. I caught my breath as the pounding of my heart eased.

When I could talk I told her, "I have never felt so good in all my life."

Mary Ellen turned on her side, her face literally glowing. "I love you, Johnny."

We embraced and gazed at the moon and stars above, lying naked in the sand, attempting to hold onto our first taste of true ecstasy.

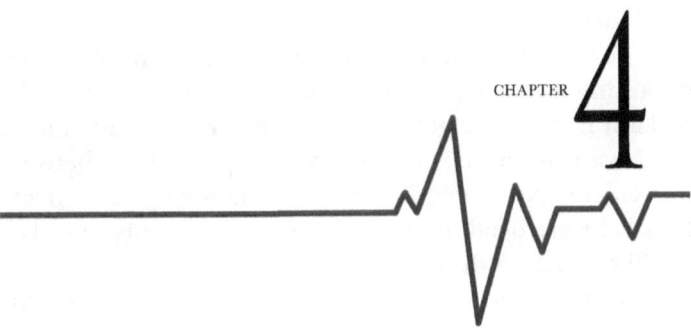

CHAPTER 4

ICU

*B*eep. *Beep. Beep.*

The portable monitor announced its approach.

"Oh, Christ, here comes Mac with the commissioner now."

"I thought someone said they would be down in CAT scan for at least an hour."

"Well, they probably did a rush job since he's the commissioner."

"Yeah, I guess. The bedside is all set, right, Mary?"

"All the emergency medicine is there and ready."

"Mr. West, we are going to move you from the stretcher into the bed now."

"Mac, is he responding at all?"

"No, Mary."

"How was the CAT scan? Did it show anything?"

"No, it was unequivocal."

"Are we ready? Okay, on the count of three. One, two—three. Jesus, watch out for his head. He almost hit the headboard."

"Sorry."

I felt my head jerk for a moment. I must have been dreaming. I was with Mary Ellen on the beach. Where the hell am I? All those voices are around again. I can't move.

I want to get up. I want to get up. Why is there no movement? No strength. Oh, God, then why can I hear? I wish I were dead; it would be better than this. If only I could go back to sleep.

"Roll him over to me first, Mary, so we can get this shit out from underneath him."

"Okay, Karen."

"Mary, his face is beginning to twitch. Jesus, it looks as though he is going to seize on us. Get Mac—now."

"Mac! Mr. West is seizing."

My body was jerking spastically; I could feel myself slipping into darkness and could no longer hear the voices again.

Lights were flashing.

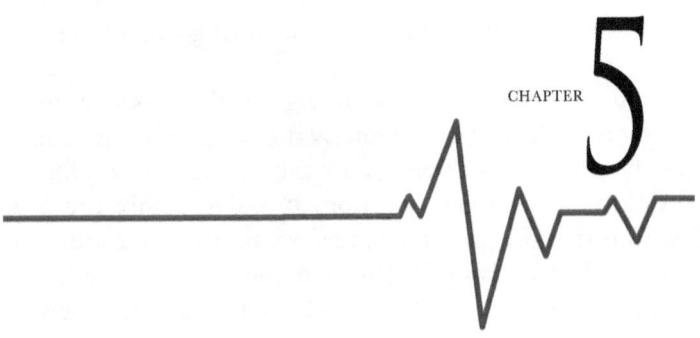

CHAPTER 5

John

Every time the dean called a name, camera flashes went off like a series of starbursts as the graduate's family excitedly captured the diploma presentation.

My big day had arrived. I was graduating summa cum laude from Harvard. Mom, Sam, and Mary Ellen were sitting proudly in the audience. I had worked so hard and was now reaping the reward. Dad would have been so honored to see his son graduate from his old alma mater. Wherever he was, I hoped he was watching this day.

"John Cameron West," the dean announced emphatically.

I strode across the stage, smiling toward the flashes. I took my diploma, shook the dean's hand, and officially left my college years behind. When the ceremony was over I joined my family, getting hugs and congratulations.

The day was also bittersweet. My roommate Bill Hadley and I had become like brothers during our time at Harvard. It was one of those magnetic friendships where you know what the other one is thinking ninety percent of the time.

Bill came from a family of eight siblings, so he knew what it was like to go without. By the same token, he ambitiously sought what was his for the taking. He was handsome and always neatly groomed and stylishly dressed. He considered himself a ladies' man, but sometimes he was a little too cocky for his own good and got stood up. It didn't bother him in the least if I told him when he was out of line.

He would always say, "Johnny, self-assertiveness will take you a long way in life. After all these years of knowing me, I hope some of it has rubbed off on you."

I understood what he meant. In the world beyond college doors, you were either an ambitious achiever or a non-aggressor who would likely fall by the wayside, waiting to be picked up.

On graduation night we went to a party at Bill's, then five years went by before I saw Bill again at our fraternity's five-year reunion. Bill had gone to law school in California, then returned to the East Coast—with his wife—and settled in Boston. He was the last person I would have expected to settle down so soon. But for all that had changed in his life, Bill was more ambitious than ever.

He quickly established himself in a law practice, always seeming to know the right door to knock. At the same time, he also managed to get himself involved in politics for the City of Boston. Most of his dealings seemed to be legal, but I questioned the ethics of the shrewd tactics he employed.

During those same five years, I received my PhD in business from Yale. I chose Yale for graduate school not only for its excellent departmental program in business but also just to get a little space. Mary Ellen was doing extremely well in Harvard's drama program, but we found it difficult to get much accomplished being around each other continuously. We had grown so close in those years at Harvard that we mutually agreed a separation would do us good and give us an opportunity to meet new people.

A month after the fraternity reunion, Bill left some urgent messages for me to call him back. After some small talk he told me he needed my help.

"What kind of help?"

"I've been kicking around city hall as a lawyer for just over a year now. You can't believe the cronyism. Down here it's *I'll kiss yours if you'll kiss mine*. I got into a little trouble because I didn't understand how it was expected to work at first. DAs want to get convictions whether the defendant is guilty or not. I've heard defense attorneys have had their families threatened to force them into convincing their clients to take a guilty plea."

"So exactly what does this all have to do with me?"

"Hold onto your pants, Johnny. I'm going to run for mayor and clean up city hall."

"I don't believe it."

"It's true."

"You don't have a snowball's chance in hell. First of all, nobody knows who you are."

"That is where you come in. With your background in business, we can have a fighting chance. And I trust you."

"I don't know, Bill. It sounds awfully far-fetched." Plus, I couldn't help but wonder what I'd be getting myself into, because I didn't completely trust my old college friend.

"Will you at least think about it? I want to right this city structure if I can."

"I'll give it some thought, but don't bank on anything. I'll get back to you."

After hanging up, I decided to fly up to New York and see Mary Ellen. She was in an actor's workshop studying for a small part in an off-off-Broadway play. After getting lost a couple of times, I finally found the street where the workshop was located in what appeared to be a sketchy neighborhood. It was on a particularly narrow street off Broadway. The sidewalks were cluttered with overflowing garbage cans and graffiti covered most of the buildings. I kept thinking: *What in the world would a theater be doing down this street?*

Walking down the street I saw a small wooden sign on the front door of a building that read: *Theater Workshop.* A man about thirty-five was leaning against the building, taking a long drag on a cigarette when I made an overture.

"Do you know if this is the theater where an off-Broadway play called *Autumn* is rehearsing?"

The man never took his eyes off the ground. "Up one flight, third door on your right."

I was hoping to surprise Mary Ellen, but the door to the rehearsal room was locked. I knocked, and the longer I stood there, the more anxious I got. Finally, after a second and much louder knock, a man with long golden hair opened the door.

"Yeah, man, what do you want?"

"I'm looking for Mary Ellen Brougham. Is she here?"

"Wait a minute," he said and shut the door.

A couple of minutes passed before he came back, and this time the distinctive aroma of marijuana came wafting through the door.

"She's not here, man."

"Do you know where she is?" I asked.

"Nope, she hasn't shown up yet."

"This is where you're rehearsing for the play *Autumn*, is it not?"

"Oh, sure, man, if that is what you were told. Are you on some kind of trip?"

Jesus, I thought, *what the hell is this?*

I turned around and started down the stairs and stopped abruptly when I saw Mary Ellen and the guy from downstairs walking up. I just stared at her.

She stared back. "Johnny! What are you doing here? I didn't expect to see you."

"I can see that, Mary Ellen."

I could hardly believe my eyes. She looked like hell. Her hair was frizzy and much longer, hanging in front of her face, which was pale and drawn. As my eyes drifted down from her face, I felt my legs become weak. She was pregnant. I was speechless.

"Surprised, Johnny?" she asked, looking me straight in the eye.

I said nothing.

"Hal," she said to the guy with her, "Go on, I'll meet you later. I want to talk to Johnny. He is an old friend."

She took my hand and led me down the stairs. We walked to a small coffee house on Broadway in silence.

My hands were shaking as I tried to drink my coffee. She began to talk about coming to New York with such high expectations of becoming an actress.

"Johnny, you know that's my dream. Well, I went nowhere. I bounced around from agency to agency, looking for bit parts. Even the bit parts were taken up by more experienced actresses."

As she talked, I realized she wasn't the same person I had known before in Boston. She seemed lost.

"Producers would soft-talk you and tell you what a fine actress you would be if you got the right part. In their offices, they had pictures of movie stars that they had supposedly given their big break to. But most were just interested in getting you on the casting couch. Then my very last agent said he knew of a small off-Broadway production called 'Autumn.' It was my final hope. The play's about the '60s—the Civil Rights Movement, the Cultural Revolution hippies, and drugs. Hal is the producer, and most of the cast is for real. They are the people from the sixties. They lived through it and have never grown out of it. I think it will become a success because of the reality of it."

"Where do you fit in?" I asked.

"Hal saw my Irish face and immediately decided that I would be the leading lady. I didn't even have to read for the part. And with my Irish Catholic background and innocence, he said it would be perfect."

"The pregnancy, is that perfect?"

She paused before replying. "No, not exactly. It was planned for the part."

"Christ, Mary Ellen, have you no conscience? That's bull about your innocence and Irish Catholic background. You're a damn hypocrite."

"I was desperate, Johnny. Have you never been desperate? My career means everything to me."

"Does life mean anything to you? Whose child is it? Don't tell me; let me guess. Hal's, right?"

She looked down. "Yes."

"Couldn't you have faked the pregnancy for the play?"

"Hal wanted everything real for the production."

"Even if it means producing a life that's not wanted? Do you love him, Mary Ellen?" She finally lifted her eyes off the table and looked me straight in the eye.

"No, Johnny, I do not love Hal."

"You've certainly changed," I told her. "You have done a complete about-face from that innocent Irish Catholic girl, as you have so deftly put it, that I once knew. How many months pregnant are you?"

"Five and a half."

"You look like eight months. What if the show is a smashing success? Are you going to continue having children regardless of who the producer is?"

"That is not fair."

"The hell it isn't," I screamed, causing everyone in the restaurant to look at us. "How the hell are you being fair to the unborn child? When it gets old enough, are you going to admit you gave them life because of a ridiculous play?"

"That's enough, Johnny. I've heard all I want to hear."

"You bet it is. I never loved anyone like I've loved you. You were my life. I thought in time we would marry and have children together. You have tossed away everything we ever had. As far as I'm concerned, we're through." I stood up. "And don't worry, I won't say a thing to your mother about this. The privilege is going to be all yours."

I looked at her face, which revealed no expression. The only visible emotion was the tears streaming from her eyes. I leaned over the table and kissed her goodbye. I walked away from that coffee house with an emptiness in my soul, thinking about the beautiful days with Mary Ellen when we were growing up.

My hurt and disappointment at losing Mary Ellen was bitter and hard to swallow. Drops of rain slid across the window as my plane made its ascent out of New York. I felt all alone and as gray as the city below, wondering if I would ever see Mary Ellen again.

———

I was deeply depressed when I got home and put off calling Bill. After much thought I contacted him at his office and gave him an abbreviated version of what had happened in New York. His reaction was one of disbelief, and it cooled his anger over me not contacting him sooner.

"Jesus, Johnny, I had no idea what you were going through. Have you told anyone else?"

"No. I don't want to hurt Mom, Sam, or anyone else. I told Mary Ellen that it would be her privilege to tell her own mother. She more than anyone won't believe what's happened. So please keep this to yourself."

"You can count on it," Bill promised. "Can you come to my office this afternoon, Johnny? Better still, why don't we meet for lunch at the Oyster House, say around one o'clock?"

"That will be fine. See you then."

As I walked down the street toward the restaurant,

people were busily going about their business. It was a clear day with a cool, crisp breeze. I could not stop thinking about Mary Ellen and if I'd had any effect on her whatsoever.

I entered the restaurant and spotted Bill at the bar. As usual he had his scotch and soda in hand.

"I didn't think you were going to make it, Johnny."

"Neither did I. That damn Volkswagen keeps stalling. It's too old to get around anymore."

"Don't worry. If your answer is yes, a new car will be provided for you. But before we get down to business, let's have lunch."

After we got a table and ordered, Bill leaned forward. "So, Johnny, what's your decision?"

"Well, I figure it like this. I'm with you all the way!"

Bill let out a loud whoop. "That's great."

Laughing, I pushed him aside. "Stop hugging me."

"Can't help it. I'm so happy. Without you, I don't think I would be able to make it happen."

"Don't count your chickens and all that," I warned him.

"I know, but I have complete trust in you. After we eat let's head over to my office and go through some of the details. By the way, if you feel like talking about Mary Ellen, I'm all ears."

"Thanks, Bill, but not right now."

We ate quickly and were soon dodging traffic crossing the street to city hall. When we arrived at Bill's office, he picked up a folder on his desk with my name on it and proceeded to explain what my duties would include.

"First off, you will be my campaign manager, my right-hand man, and most important, my confidant. You will be aware of everything that is taking place throughout the campaign. When Aunt Maggie from Connecticut died, she left me quite a bit of money. I suppose she left it to me because she knew I was running for councilman.

"So whatever you need, Johnny, money will not be a problem. If you feel you need to hire extras, your judgment is fine with me. I want you to have free rein with this campaign. Your integrity and honesty are binding."

"I'm glad you feel that way. I'll do my best."

"That's enough for me."

We parted with a firm handshake and an agreement to have our next meeting in two weeks. I took home a multitude of papers to develop a schedule for Bill, prepare a candidacy announcement, and work on strategies to start his campaign. It wasn't as easy as I thought it would be, but in two weeks' time I had set up a campaign headquarters in downtown Boston.

It was a lucky break because it was situated right in the heart of the business district, a high-traffic area. Satellite headquarters were set up in nine of the eleven districts on the periphery. I wanted to give Bill as much publicity as possible. Only honest-to-goodness hard workers were hired for this campaign, which meant volunteering long hours and most weekends. It wasn't all hard work; we had lots of fun too.

We had *Hadley for Mayor* printed on every kind of merchandise we could think of—buttons, hats, bumper stickers, combs, and even fingernail files. I had spent a lot of money, but I knew he would be pleased.

Finally, Bill's big day arrived as we celebrated the opening of his headquarters in Boston, which coincided with him officially announcing his mayoral candidacy. Bill arrived with his pregnant wife, Liz, at about 5:00 p.m. When he opened the door and looked in at all the people clapping for him, with his name adorned everywhere, tears trickled from his eyes. He came over and gave me the tightest bear hug that I thought would crack my ribs.

"Johnny, I'm speechless. I don't believe you were able to do all this in just two weeks."

Bill made his way to the podium to say a few words. "I'm not going to make a speech tonight, but Liz and I want to express heartfelt thanks to everyone who made this possible. And listen up—dinner is on me! Everyone is invited to the Skylight Tower Restaurant after the reception here ends. The celebration will mark the beginning of my mayoral campaign."

With applause and loud cheers, everyone gave Bill a champagne toast, already calling him Mayor Hadley. I had to warn him not to let it go to his head.

The Skylight Tower Restaurant resides in one of the tallest buildings in Boston, overlooking the city's skyline. Everyone was drinking champagne and thoroughly enjoying themselves at the restaurant. It was a great idea of Bill's, and it complemented the respect we all had for him.

Conversation flowed as we were immersed in our main course. I looked up from my shrimp scampi to see a waiter approach the table and hand Bill a piece of paper. When Bill read the note, his face went white. I casually suggested to Bill that we get some fresh air. Once out on the terrace, Bill handed me the note.

It read: *You better drop out of this race or else!*

"Who in the hell would have sent this, Johnny?" Bill asked, sounding frightened. "I only officially announced my campaign tonight."

"That's true, but it was all over town that you were going to run for mayor. It's probably just a prank," I said with more confidence than I felt. "You go on back inside so no one gets suspicious, and I'll try to find out who gave the note to the waiter."

I found the waiter in the lounge. I grabbed his arm, and after coaxing him with a $20 bill, he told me a young teenage kid about five-foot-six and wearing a jogging suit had handed him the note and told him to give it to Bill Hadley.

"Did he say anything else?"

"No. That was all he asked me to do."

I drove Bill and Liz home to see them safely to the door. Bill had been lost in thought the entire way home, and before he got out of the car, he told me he was going to drop out of the race.

"I think it's too risky to run. I have to think of everyone's safety in all this."

"Look, Bill, you cannot back down anytime someone threatens you. You don't even know if the note is for real."

"Real or not, Johnny, what if they go after my family?"

"We have enough money to put a guard around the clock on Liz. Whoever it is, they don't want you to get the slightest piece of the action. To back out now is what they want. Don't you see that? Besides, you want more than anything to become mayor of this town, right?"

"You don't even have to ask that," Bill said. "I just don't want to jeopardize anyone's safety."

"Let's take this one step at a time, and if we get any more threats, the police will be brought in on it," I assured him. "We'll post guards around the clock on your family and anyone who has a major dealing with the campaign."

"I guess you're right. That seems to be the most sensible thing to do. No use jumping the gun." He put his hand on my shoulder. "I'm sure glad to have you as my friend through all of this."

I nodded and smiled. "Listen, you two get some sleep, and I'll call you first thing in the morning."

They got out, and before shutting the door, Bill said, "Be careful on the way home."

"Right."

I must admit, I kept looking in the rearview mirror the entire drive home. I was thinking of how quiet and reserved Liz had been throughout our conversation. If she had said she was scared, especially being pregnant, Bill would have dropped out of the race for her. I admired Liz's guts.

A few days later we heard that Jack Rizzo was also entering the race for mayor. He was a well-known Italian from the north end of Boston. The reason Rizzo was so notable was because of his assets in real estate and his alleged involvement in organized crime. Bill brought up the possibility that it may have been Rizzo who was behind the note.

"It's sure a possibility," I agreed.

"He's been wheeling and dealing down here at city hall for many a year."

"Yeah, but why all of a sudden is he going to run for mayor?"

"I don't know, Johnny. Maybe the gang is in trouble and needs help through the city. It could be for any number of reasons, but it will definitely take votes away from me, that I know for sure."

"What do you think of putting a tail on him?"

Bill shook his head. "Sounds risky, and what would we gain from it?"

"It might give us an edge as to why all of a sudden he's going to run for mayor. With that information we could certainly strengthen our strategy."

"We're not fooling around with high school kids, Johnny. If Rizzo ever found out, his people usually don't give a warning. They'd just as soon pop you as look at you."

"I know, and I have reservations," I admitted. "But if we want to win, it's a chance we're going to have to take. Do I have your permission to do it?"

After much hesitation, Bill nodded. "Put someone on it you know you can trust. Make sure they are as discreet as possible."

"I have just the man in mind."

"Really? Who?"

"Do you remember Ken Reed from the newspaper?"

"Vaguely. The columnist?"

"That's right. He's not only a good friend of mine, but he also does impressions, complete with makeup and costumes for the kids down at the Ronald McDonald House. He's really terrific with those kids. He makes them smile and laugh through their illness."

"He sounds like quite a person."

"He certainly is. I'll get in touch with him tonight and feel him out. It'll be a dangerous assignment, but who knows, maybe there will be a meaty story in it for him."

"Just as long as he's aware of the danger and doesn't get himself killed in the process," Bill said.

"Not this kid. He's extremely careful, and if I know Ken, he'll be in a different disguise every time he's out on patrol. Do you know the other two candidates?

"Fairly well. One is the former school chairman, John O'Keefe, and the other is Ted Wagner, who's also on the council. They're both hard-working men with damn good track records. It'll be a difficult race."

"Well, then, I better get busy on some of those speeches and appearance dates. See you soon, Bill."

"Soon" ended up being three days. I had a lot of catching up to do as well as some nosing around. When I finally showed up at Bill's office, he wasn't pleased.

"Where in the hell have you been for three days, Johnny? I've been trying to reach you."

"Don't be too upset; I was just checking up on a few matters."

"Such as?"

"Well, Ken Reed agreed to follow Rizzo."

"He's aware of the potential danger, is he not?"

"I didn't have to warn him at all. Apparently, Ken has had dealings indirectly with him before. Ken's uncle was involved with the numbers in South Boston about fifteen years ago. The way Ken remembers it, his uncle had taken over the business for a friend named Paulo, who was Rizzo's cousin. They were old-timers, and it didn't matter to them about ethnic backgrounds or the gang. They were good friends that could trust one another, and that was their only concern.

"When Paulo died, he left his entire share of their business to Ken's uncle. However, when Rizzo's father heard about this, all hell broke loose. He somehow expected it to go to one of his own.

"To make a long but sad story short, one day Ken's uncle was driving home from the grocery store. As he was waiting at a stop sign, a black sedan pulled up alongside his car and let him have it in broad daylight. Can you imagine that? He was an old man and probably wouldn't have had the business very long anyway."

Bill looked worried. "I don't know if this is going to work. It sounds as if he's too personally involved. I don't want to see anyone get hurt just because of a campaign."

"I can understand that. But involved or not, he knows why we're going to put a tail on Rizzo. He wants the assignment. Besides, he's too careful and prudent."

"I hope you're right."

"On other matters, I've composed some of your speeches and arranged a list of appearances that you can look over. Have you been working on a proposed budget plan?"

"Partially. I'm still trying to lower taxes while also reducing the city's budget. It's tough, but if I can work on some of the hierarchy's overpaid salaries, I think I can do it."

I smiled at Bill. "Just don't put that last part into writing until you're in. Some of the big issues this year that the people need to hear about are busing, lowering taxes, inflation, oil prices, and housing for the elderly. You wouldn't believe the number of old people that died last year because of no heat."

Bill put his hand up, not in the mood for a campaign lecture. "I know all that."

"Okay. Family and community involvement will certainly be a plus as well. When is Liz due?"

"Around the end of October."

"That'll be great, just before the election. Pictures of you, Liz, and the new baby will represent a solid family unit."

"Why don't we continue this discussion at dinner at my house tonight?" Bill suggested. "You really haven't spent much time around Liz, and it would be a good opportunity before all the commotion starts. Besides, she'd love it."

"So would I."

"Is six o'clock okay?"

"That will be fine. See you then."

I left wondering if Bill could really win the election. My gut feeling was that he had a damn good chance. My next stop was a quick meeting with Ken. Over coffee he said that so far, Rizzo hadn't done anything, nor had he seen anyone suspicious, but he would stay on him, believing it was only a matter of time.

I went back to my office at the campaign headquarters to work on some things, then walked to Bill and Liz's for dinner. They were renting the most beautiful apartment on Beacon Hill. It was spacious with a winding staircase up to the master bedroom, which boasted a fireplace and a large picture window that overlooked the city.

The night was clear, the stars shimmered in the sky, and it felt good to be alive and able to absorb it all. When I approached Bill's front door and rang the bell, it had a unique tone to it. I wondered if it was the original bell that was installed when the apartment was built.

Bill answered the door and ushered me into the living room, where Liz and another woman were sitting. Liz said hello and then introduced me.

"Johnny, I would like you to meet a good friend of mine, Linda Haynes. Linda, this is my husband's best friend, Johnny West."

"Glad to meet you," I said.

"Same here."

"Linda is in fashion design. Not only is she planning to open her own shop, but a school as well."

"Don't jump the gun, Liz. If everything goes well financially, I'll hopefully be able to open up soon."

"Where do you plan to open your school?" I asked.

"You know that old building on the corner of Newbury and Dartmouth? I put a bid into the city to buy it so I can restore it. It's got so much history and character. Of course, they practically laughed in my face, so I established some plans with my brother who, luckily, is an architect. We presented my plan to the Building Commission and the Historical Society and finally got it approved. Now, if I can just get the loan approved from the bank, I'll be in business."

"That sounds terrific," I said.

I found myself caught up with her graciousness and beauty. It was soon obvious that Bill and Liz were trying to play cupid. Between the campaign and my own broken heart, I had not dated since Mary Ellen. I had to admit that Linda certainly was beautiful, cerebral, and a perfect lady.

Dinner was lively with conversation and laughter. We had just finished when an explosion of shattering glass had us jumping out of our chairs and running toward the front room, where the window was smashed to pieces.

"What the hell ..." I looked outside but saw nobody.

Linda pointed. "Look over there," she said with an ominous tone in her voice.

There was a medium-sized rock on the floor with a piece of paper tied to it. Bill walked over and picked it up.

"What's the note say," I asked.

This is a second warning. There will be no third warning. Get out of the race while you're still alive.

Bill raised up his fist in anger. "I'll kill the son of a bitch who's doing this."

"Cool down," I told him. "Let's think this through."

Bill glared at me. "How can you be so damn calm about this?"

"That's what they want. They want us angry and afraid. Yes, I'll admit, I am a little scared, but I'm a lot determined not to let them intimidate me. We can do something about this."

"I don't know, Johnny," Liz said. "First the note at the restaurant, and now another one hurled through our window. Lord knows what's next. I'm scared."

Bill tried to comfort her, his expression reflecting his own fear.

I reminded him, "We promised each other if this should happen again, the police would be brought in."

"Do you think it's wise?"

"Yes, Bill, I do. It's the only sensible thing to do right now."

I went to the phone, placed a call to the station, and asked for Sergeant Buckley. As soon as he got on the phone, I heard the concern in his voice.

"I've been trying to reach you for the past hour."

"Why? What's wrong?"

"Ken Reed was stabbed about an hour ago, and he's been asking for you."

"Sergeant, would you be able to come over to Bill Hadley's house? We have had some trouble over here, too."

"Is anyone hurt?"

"No, but I think it's important that you get here as soon as possible."

"Okay, see you in about twenty minutes."

After I hung up I told Bill what had happened to Ken.

"I knew something like this was going to happen," he said, his voice clipped. "I told you. Is he all right?"

"He's awake and asking for me."

"Let's go see him right now."

"Wait, Bill. The police are on their way here right now.

As soon as they get here, we can go. I don't think it's wise to leave you until we have protection in place. From now until this election is over, everyone concerned will have security."

"This is getting really dirty."

"I know, but we just need to go about our business. The election is only three months away. Everything we do will be on a need-to-know basis."

"And I'll stay out of the picture," Liz said. "No personal appearances, no interviews, no showing up at headquarters. We can just tell people I'm on bed rest, doctor's orders."

Linda nodded. "As long as they think she's not participating in the campaign, the better it'll be for her."

"Okay, but the security stays," Bill said. "I'm not taking any chances."

Linda was watching the street from behind the curtain, waiting for the police. It seemed as though it was taking them forever to get there, but it had probably only been a few minutes since I'd hung up with Buckley.

"Here they are!" she said with a relieved look on her face.

"Thank God!" I muttered and went to open the front door. "Sergeant Buckley, I'm glad you are here."

"I wish it weren't under these circumstances, Johnny."

He examined the rock and note closely. "We'll try to lift fingerprints, but if it has anything to do with the gang I believe is behind this, we won't find any evidence."

After bagging the rock and handing it to another officer, Buckley turned to Bill. "We are putting together protection details."

"Thank you, Sergeant. Do you have any leads on Ken Reed yet?"

"I'm afraid not. He's in surgery for some internal bleeding. They may have to remove his spleen and repair part of his bowel."

"Do they think he'll pull through?" Bill asked.

"He lost a lot of blood, but they told me that his chances were pretty good."

"I guess there's no point in going down there to try and see him then," I said.

"No, he won't be out of surgery for hours, then will be in recovery. Guards will be posted outside his door twenty-four hours a day."

"Okay. Do you know exactly what happened?"

"Well, we have one witness who said Ken came out of the Oyster House restaurant across from city hall about seven o'clock. She said just before he crossed the street, two men jumped out of a blue car and attacked him. She didn't know the make and model and didn't get the plate number. We don't know if Ken will be able to make a positive identification or not, but once he regains consciousness from surgery, we'll find out. Hopefully, he will regain consciousness."

"If I know Ken, he'll give it every last breath he has to fight back," I said with confidence.

After going over the logistics of the security details, I asked Linda if she wanted to share a cab to our respective homes.

"I'd appreciate it."

Before saying our goodnights, Bill pulled me aside. "Do you think Rizzo knew Ken was on his tail?"

"Sure looks like it."

"Christ, I wish I had never agreed to it."

"Don't blame yourself. Ken is an expert at surveillance. Something had to slip up. What, we won't know until he's conscious. So get some sleep, and in the morning we'll get some answers."

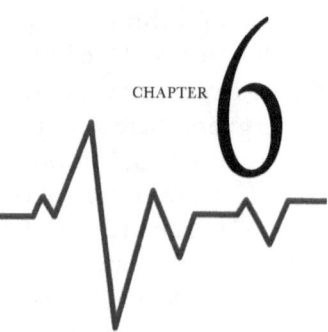

John

Ken suffered some complications, so it was three weeks before we talked to him. I gathered from Sergeant Buckley that the police had no leads whatsoever. They never found the car, and the description they had of the men involved was too vague for any positive identification.

I always found hospitals somewhat ominous, with their starched white decor and the distinctive odor of alcohol cleansers. I hadn't been near a hospital since Dad was ill, and that was some time ago. I felt all those memories coming back to me when Bill and I stepped off the elevator and approached the room.

Ken was sitting up in bed, and I thought he looked like a skeleton waiting to be boxed to a medical school.

"Good to see you, Ken," Bill said. "We thought we were going to lose you."

"I know. It was touch and go for a while."

"You've lost so much weight," I said. "How do you really feel?"

"Well, I don't think I'm up for a marathon, but my appetite is coming back, and each day I walk a little farther and feel a little stronger. Never mind about me. How's the campaign going?"

"Very well," Bill said. "We have a damn good chance at it. My speeches are going over well, and with the publicity of your incident, I don't think the public will be too quick to trust Rizzo. Even though there's been no direct connection to him in the newspapers, there are suggestions hinting as much. Do you remember anything about the incident?"

Ken shook his head. "I've gone over it in my head a thousand times. I had just come out of the restaurant and was about to cross the street. After that, everything is a total blackout until I woke up in the hospital. The doctors said it was from getting hit in the head. What do you make of it, Johnny?"

"The way I figure it, they were astute enough to pick up that someone was tailing them."

"I know that if it leaked out that I was tailing them for Bill, it wouldn't look good for his campaign."

"Well, it's all over," I told him. "In retrospect, it was a stupid idea. What's important is that you're alive and getting well. That's all that counts."

"I'll be out of here in no time."

"I hope so." Bill patted his shoulder. "However, from now on in, you'll be protected through the campaign, even though you don't have anything to do with it."

"Won't that create suspicion?"

"It shouldn't," I assured him. "Like I said, there are undertones that Rizzo indeed had something to do with it."

"Well, I hope I'll be able to visit from time to time."

"Of course, Ken, without question," Bill said, glancing at his watch.

"We better be on our way," I told Ken. "I'll stop by in a couple of days."

"Okay, Johnny."

As Bill and I left the hospital, I wondered if Ken would ever be the same again after going through such a traumatic experience. I only had myself to blame for asking him to follow Rizzo.

We went back to Bill's office to go over what needed to be taken care of while he was out of town. He and Liz were going to Texas for a week to see her family. In addition to taking a break, Bill thought it best to be away for a short while and let things calm down.

Once we finished and he was getting ready to leave, Bill handed me a piece of paper.

"I want you to have Liz's parent's phone number in case anything comes up."

"Thanks. But I want you to just concentrate on relaxing and enjoy the time away. When you get back, you're going to have a very tight schedule. So, go and forget about all the problems up here for the next week."

"Thanks, Johnny. I really appreciate this. Have you heard from Mary Ellen?"

"No, I haven't heard from her, but I've heard *about* her. I ran into her mother about a week ago. Apparently, she hadn't heard from Mary Ellen in more than eight months. From what her mother tells me, she's doing quite well. That play she was in was an enormous success, and it's been uphill since then."

"Is she happy?"

I shrugged. "She's living out in California now, getting roles in movies. So I really don't know if she's happy or not, but she's successful, which is what she always wanted."

"I'm sorry it didn't work out for the two of you."

"Don't be. I'm not doing so bad myself since you introduced me to a wonderful girl."

Bill looked surprised. "Are you and Linda dating now?"

"We have been since shortly after dinner at your place that night."

"I think that's great. I knew you would hit it off. I was getting worried about you. After Mary Ellen, you practically became a recluse."

"It's all behind me now."

He paused at the door. "Call if you need me for anything."

"Give Liz my best, and I'll see you both in a week or so. Now go."

It was quiet the week Bill was away. There were no more threats, no drama of any kind. I saw Ken again, and he was starting to look like his old self again. I saw Linda as much as our schedules would allow us.

———

Easter was coming up. Thursday night, after wrapping things up in Bill's office, I called Linda to ask her if she'd like to go to Vermont for the weekend. She said yes immediately. With the campaign heating up, I knew my schedule would be getting busy, so it was a good opportunity for some time together.

We left early Friday morning, bubbling with joy like two kids. We took our time getting there, stopping at shops and wherever we pleased as we drove. We stayed at the famous Greenwood Inn in northern Vermont. Spring was just making its appearance, and the days were getting warmer, now in the mid-fifties with clear skies the entire weekend. The Inn had everything to offer: tennis, golf, swimming, horseback riding, and fishing.

We were so thrilled to be away that I completely forgot about the campaign. Linda and I went for long walks through the countryside, sharing about our pasts, including old loves and how they had affected our lives. Up to then I had been hesitant to discuss my relationship with Mary Ellen. But as we approached one of Vermont's oldest covered bridges that spanned a babbling brook that drained into a small river, I decided it was time, in this idyllic spot, to finally discuss my hurt. Linda listened quietly as I told her about Mary Ellen, what she had meant to me, and how it ended. When I finished, I asked Linda about her first love.

"Well, to make a long story short, when I was about fifteen, naive, and gullible, there was a boy who lived in the next town over. His name was Charley Murphy. He was a year older and came from a very wealthy family. Looking back now I can see he had the charm of a snake, but I fell head over heels for him.

"One day he asked me if I would like to see the guest house, which was about one hundred yards behind the main house. I knew something was off because as soon as we went inside, he locked the door. And then his whole personality changed. He came at me like an animal and raped me."

"God, Linda, I'm so sorry."

"It was my own stupid fault."

"That's nonsense. You were in no way culpable. Did you call the police?"

"No. But I finally told my father, and he was furious. He said if it took his last breath, Murphy would pay for what he did. To everyone's surprise, with my father's ranting and raving about it, more and more came out in the open. Apparently, he had done the same thing to a half dozen other girls before me."

"Nothing was done to him? How could that be?" I asked. "Didn't his parents do anything about it?"

"My father pressed for charges and got support from all the other parents. But Charley's parents sent him away to a psychiatric hospital, and somehow he was never charged."

"What happened to him?"

"He's now a well-known psychiatrist with a very successful practice."

"I cannot believe they would let him go into such a field."

"He has money, Johnny, and money buys power."

———

That night we went into Woodstock for dinner at a small restaurant named Jenny's, owned by a good friend of my mother. Before heading to the restaurant, I took Linda on a tour of the town. She was thrilled with its boutiques and the general store where you could purchase anything from soup to nuts.

It was just about dusk when we arrived at Jenny's and were greeted by the redolent aroma from the two wood stoves burning day and night in the restaurant. It was the most popular spot in town and with good reason.

The interior was pine wood braced with solid oak beams and looked like a scene out of the old frontier. There was sawdust on the floor with both booths and small tables for intimate dining. Hanging plants were evenly distributed in every window.

We sat at a table near one of the wood stoves. Linda took a long look around, contemplating the atmosphere.

"The restaurant is everything you said it would be," she said.

"Do you see those old guns in that case by the entrance? They were Jenny's father's when he was in the war. They're probably worth a lot of money today. There's Jenny now. Excuse me."

I approached Jenny from behind and gave her a hug. "Guess who?"

She spun around on her heels. "Johnny West! Well, I'll be doggone. Come over here in the light and let me get a good look at you. Hmm, you're as handsome as ever."

"You never stop flattering, do you, Jenny?"

"Not when it comes to you. Is everything all right at home?"

"Everything is good. Mom is in the best of health. And I'm up here to relax before the campaign gets into full throttle."

"Your mother wrote to me about the campaign. She's worried."

"We don't anticipate any more trouble."

"I hope not. Now, are you going to introduce me to that lovely young lady looking our way?"

"I'm terribly sorry." I brought her over to our table. "Jenny McDuffie, this is Linda Haynes."

After they exchanged hellos, Jenny gestured toward the menus. "Do you know what you want?"

I smiled. "I'll have the usual."

"Johnny, one day you must try something besides the beef stroganoff."

"No one makes it like you do."

"Well, then, make it two orders of beef stroganoff," Linda said.

"It'll be ready in about twenty minutes."

A few moments later, our waiter brought us a bottle of very nice wine. "Compliments of the house," he said.

Jenny continued to spoil us throughout the entire meal, catering to our every wish. The hot, homemade rolls that melted in your mouth arrived at the table first. The beef stroganoff was superb, served with tender tips of asparagus steamed to perfection. The pièce de résistance was the homemade apple pie for dessert. We savored every last morsel.

After we finished eating, Jenny was able to visit us for a moment.

"Did you enjoy yourself?"

"Jenny, dinner was magnificent," I said.

"Good. If you don't mind, Johnny, would you give this to your mom?"

She held out an envelope. "Certainly." I took the envelope and put it in my jacket pocket, then stood to hug her goodnight. "The next time I come up, I'll bring Mom with me."

"That would be wonderful."

Jenny embraced me tightly, then she turned to Linda. "It was truly a pleasure to have met you. I hope to see you again."

"You can count on it," Linda promised.

We left a short time later and walked back to the inn under the moonlight arm in arm, breathing in the beautiful evening. I couldn't remember the last time I felt so wonderfully relaxed.

We arrived at the inn around eleven o'clock and sat out on the porch. I felt myself drawing closer and closer to Linda, and her to me. Sunday was approaching too fast. I wished I could somehow stop time.

We said goodnight a little after midnight. I went to my room, longing for her to come with me. It would have been the perfect ending to a perfect night. But if she wasn't ready, I would wait.

I was about to get under the covers when there was a soft knock on the door.

"Johnny, it's Linda."

I opened the door to find Linda standing there in a long, diaphanous nightgown. I swept her up into my arms, and our lips never parted as I carried her to the bed. It was an enchanted night.

The following morning I lay watching Linda sleeping and knew I had fallen in love.

No sooner had those thoughts entered my mind when her eyes opened. She rolled on top of me with a shout of joy.

"I didn't think I could ever feel love again. You make me so happy."

We kissed and caressed each other with the utmost gentleness. We were both very much in love and expressed it with words and touch and pleasure—until the maid knocked on the door because it was checkout time. We made it downstairs just in time to have breakfast, which tasted superb. Everything seemed so beautiful; I wasn't ready to leave.

"How about going horseback riding before we leave this afternoon?"

"That is a wonderful idea, Johnny. I haven't been riding for a long time. I'll probably be a little rusty."

"That makes two of us."

A little rusty wasn't the proper description for me—I almost fell off the horse twice. But it was fun. After our ride we visited the covered bridge, which had become our favorite spot, and had a picnic. We finally got on the road about four o'clock that afternoon, sad to be leaving but excited at what the future might hold.

———

I overslept the next morning and was late getting to the office. To my surprise, Bill was already there.

"How was your trip to Texas?" I asked.

"Very restful, thanks. I came back a day early to get a start on things. Was there any trouble while I was gone?"

"No, everything has been quiet. No notes or threats."

"I hope it stays that way."

"I don't think Rizzo would dare try any more assaults."

"I still don't trust Rizzo worth a damn. How is Ken doing?"

"He's looking like a human being again."

"Thank God," Bill said with a relieved sigh. "If he had died, I would have never forgiven myself."

"Well, he didn't. So right now all your energies need to be focused on getting elected mayor of this city."

"I know. I've been looking over the schedule."

"You'll have about three appearances a day. Liz isn't going to see very much of you in the next few months."

He nodded. "So how are you doing?"

"I think I am in love," I confessed.

A grin broke out on Bill's face. "You and Linda? That's great news."

"It just happened. We went to Vermont this weekend. I haven't felt this way for a long time. It's the most wonderful feeling in the world. Remember Jenny McDuffie?"

"Isn't she a friend of your mother?"

"Her dearest friend. Jenny has a restaurant in Woodstock that has the best homemade food you've ever tasted. After the election, you ought to take Liz up there for a few days; it would renew your souls."

I tried to explain how magical the restaurant had been for Linda and me. "It's like it created a magnetic closeness between us, and the rest is history. Anyway, you're speaking in front of the city union workers at two o'clock. Here's a copy of your speech. Make sure you emphasize better negotiations with the city and increased wages along with the usual proposals of health benefits, vacations, etc."

"Don't worry; I'll give it my best."

After Bill left I spent the rest of the morning working, then in the afternoon I went to deliver Jenny's letter. I found my mom sweeping the kitchen floor.

"Mom, you will never change," I teased, then shared a long hug with her. I loved that woman so much.

"Where have you been? I haven't seen you in weeks."

"Well, I didn't want to come around so soon after the trouble with Ken, just in case I was being followed. You understand, right?"

"I don't know if I'll ever understand it at all."

"The less said, the better, but I do have some good news for you," I said, changing the subject to something happier. "I've met a wonderful girl. Her name is Linda Haynes, and she's a fashion designer with her own school. She's bright, down-to-earth, pretty, and has a great personality. We went up to Vermont this weekend and had a great time."

"I have hoped and prayed you would find someone again."

"And I did. Would it be all right to bring Linda to dinner here sometime this week?"

"I would love to meet her, Johnny. Is Wednesday okay?"

"Let me call and confirm it with Linda. The other thing is Linda and I had dinner at Jenny's restaurant Saturday, and she gave me a letter for you." I handed her the envelope.

"That's really a coincidence because I was just thinking about her the other day." She put the broom away and headed toward the living room. "Would you put some coffee on for us?"

"Sure, Mom."

I had no sooner plugged in the coffee pot when I heard her crying. I hurried into the living room and found Mom in her favorite high-backed chair with the letter in her hand, her face wet with tears.

"What is it, Mom?"

She handed me the letter.

> Dear Kate,
>
> I felt that writing this news might be a little easier than if I had called you on the phone. I've been feeling so tired lately and unable to keep weight on. So I went to old Doc Sanborn, who found lumps in my breasts and sent me to the hospital for some tests.
>
> The biopsy result showed the masses were malignant, and the damn stuff had already spread throughout my body. They feel it's too far gone for any treatment and won't predict how long I have. I've lived a good life, and I'm sure the hereafter cannot be any worse.
>
> I would like for you and Johnny to come up to

Vermont and spend some time. I want to discuss what to do with the restaurant with you both.

I hope you'll forgive me for writing this way, but it was the best way I knew to tell you. I'll call you in a couple of days.

God bless, I love you.

Jenny

"Oh, Mom. I noticed Jenny had lost weight but didn't think much of it. She was her usual busy self, running all over. Why does that damn cancer strike the best of people?"

"I don't know, but it does seem that way." She wiped away her tears and sat up straight. "I'm not going to wait for her to call. I'll call her this evening and set up a date when we can go to Vermont."

"Make it soon, Mom."

I went back to the office for some appointments that took up the rest of the afternoon. When I was finally finished, I called Linda, and we agreed to meet at my place. When she arrived, I filled her in on the news about Jenny.

"How can that be? She worked feverishly around the restaurant and looked so well. Where does it go from here?"

"That's difficult to say. I think it's just one of those situations where you take it one step at a time. She wants my mom and me to go visit her and help her decide what to do with the restaurant."

"Who do you think might take it over?"

"Probably her nephew."

Linda's eyes teared. "This is so sad."

"I know. It's a slap-in-the-face reminder that no tomorrow is guaranteed. None of us know how much time we have. That's why we shouldn't waste a single day." I slid off the couch onto my knee. "I know we haven't been together long, but I'm in love with you. Will you marry me?"

Gobsmacked, Linda put a hand to her heart. "I sure didn't see that coming."

"Do you love me, Linda?"

"Yes, but it's all so fast. What's the rush?"

"I want our wedding at the Greenwood Inn and the reception at Jenny's while she's still in fair health. Plus, you're who I want, and I don't want to wait to start our life together."

Linda looked me in the eye for a long moment, then took my hand. "While it's faster than I thought it would happen, I'm in love with you too, so I'm all for it."

We kissed, then I asked, "Will you stay with me tonight?"

"If you insist."

"Oh, I do, I do."

———

The following morning, I floated into the campaign headquarters, still on cloud nine. Bill was there in our office. He stared at me.

"What has got you in such a happy mood this morning?"

"You're not going to believe this one."

"Lately, I'll believe anything."

"I'll have you know that you're the first to hear this. Linda and I are getting married."

Bill blinked at me in stunned silence for a second. "You're kidding," he said at last.

"No, it's true."

"Well, congratulations. But how come so sudden?"

A little of my joy faded. "My mom's friend Jenny is dying of cancer. I'd like to get married at the inn we just stayed at and have the reception at Jenny's restaurant while she's still healthy enough to enjoy it. It'll mean a lot to my mom too."

"That's really compassionate of you both."

"Jenny is a wonderful person, and I want to add any happiness to her life I can."

Bill nodded, then said, "Have you set an official date yet?"

"No, but it'll probably be in two or three weeks."

"I wish you all the happiness. Liz is going to be thrilled when I tell her."

"I know. Will you be my best man?"

Bill grinned. "I thought you would never ask. I'd be honored."

"I think Linda is going to ask Liz to be her matron of honor," I added.

"She'll love it."

"We'll have a splendid time then. I'll be back in a couple of hours. I need to run some errands, and I want to go see my mom."

"Take the rest of the day off. I'm all set for the day."

"Thanks, I think I will. By the way, how did that speech go over at the union workers' meeting?"

"Just great. I heard overtones that Rizzo is going to be a big loser because of the incident with Ken Reed."

"Really?"

Bill nodded. "Apparently, it's had a much bigger effect than we anticipated."

I pumped my fist. "We're going to win this race."

"I hope so."

"I know so."

Everything was looking up.

———

Linda and I set our wedding date for Saturday, May 2nd. We hoped that despite the short notice our close family and friends would all be able to attend. We arrived on Friday and were surprised by my brother Sam, who had flown in from California where he was a successful neurologist. I still couldn't believe my little brother was a doctor. He never changed in my eyes. He was his usual self, endlessly curious about the world around him. Mom was thrilled to have him around for a couple of days.

Our wedding was resplendent. Everyone enjoyed themselves immensely, and we couldn't have asked for a better day. Jenny was completely astounded that we pulled it off so quickly. I cannot remember ever seeing her so content and relaxed. Her only close relative still living was her brother, who was now eighty years old. He attended the wedding and was the life of the party with his sharp wit and love of dancing.

We stayed in Vermont for a couple of days following the wedding to spend time with Mom and Jenny. Although he wanted to stay, physician duty required Sam to get back to the West Coast.

Linda and I honeymooned for a week in the Virgin Islands, which was enchanting. We stayed at a small guest house near a marina that overlooked the ocean. The view was spectacular. On one side there was ocean as far as the eye could see; on the other were magnificent yachts and sailing vessels from all over the world coming in and out of the harbor.

We were lost in love, engulfed by the fantasy of it all. The crystal-clear waters enabled us to go snorkeling and view all kinds of small luminescent fish with the most beautiful yellow, red, blue, and purple colors. To top it all off, they were surrounded by a background of red and pink coral and ventilated by sea fans that swayed back and forth with the movement of the current.

When we arrived back from the Caribbean, there was a phone message waiting for me from my mother to call her at Jenny's as soon as I got in. I could feel my heart pound as I quickly looked for Jenny's number in the Rolodex.

My mom answered after the first ring. "I just this minute arrived back from the Caribbean and got your message. What's wrong?"

"It's Jenny. You weren't even gone two days when she experienced terrific pain in her head. I took her to the hospital, and they ran some tests. They found a tumor on the right side of her brain. Within hours she slipped into a coma, and the doctor doesn't know how long she'll live."

"I'm so sorry, Mom. I'll come up there as soon as I can."

"Hurry, Johnny."

Linda had to stay in Boston because of work, so I went to Vermont that evening by myself. By the time I arrived Jenny wasn't responding at all, and Mom looked like all the life had drained out of her too. Jenny was slipping away by the day. I'd sit beside her bed, holding her hand, and think of all the good times we shared. I was so thankful that Linda and I had decided to get married when we did, so Jenny was able to share that with us.

Her body finally gave up, and she died peacefully after sunset on May 18th. I think Mom felt relieved that Jenny's suffering was over. She was buried on the mountainside facing Woodstock, her hometown, so the sun would shine with her always.

We stayed a few days after the funeral to help her brother get back to his daily routine. His eldest son, who was a fine young man, took over the restaurant. She requested in her will that it never change, and he honored her wishes when he took it over, handling it with the utmost care, just as she wanted. With everything settled, Mom and I finally left to pick up our own lives, taking our treasured memories of Jenny with us.

In the months that followed, I was consumed with the campaign. Our progress was incredible. The local polls showed Bill as the leading mayoral candidate, so he was on a constant high. I would laugh and tease him that he had Liz to thank; people paid more attention to her pregnant belly than they did to his speeches, and he knew it.

Despite the incident with Ken Reed, Rizzo was still Bill's closest opponent and theoretically had a chance to pull an upset and win. However, in my mind he had blown his chance a long time ago by trying to scare people with war-game tactics. We continued with undercover police protection.

Linda and I moved into a new condominium complex overlooking the Charles River. Our unit was on the nineteenth floor and had a magnificent view, especially at sunset in the summertime. You could see the sailboats dance over the small crests of water as they moved slowly through the water. At night we could see the lights of the entire city.

I had never felt more relaxed and comfortable than I did on our first night above the city, gazing out the windows for hours. It became a ritual release for me after a long day of campaigning and meeting people all day long. In some ways I couldn't wait for the election to finally be over. It seemed as though we'd been campaigning for years.

We all began to feel the pressure as the end neared. A week before the election the cool, calm collectedness that Bill had always bragged about began to fray, and he was frequently a bit hotheaded and unreasonable. Everyone attributed it to the election, although I thought there were other things upsetting him.

The night of the election finally arrived. So did fatherhood. Two hours before the polls closed, Liz went into labor. Bill was torn and hesitated to leave headquarters.

"There's no need for you to hang around here," I told him.

"I guess you're right. Meet us over at the hospital after it becomes final, one way or another."

"You bet."

Bill paused at the door. "It's finally happening, isn't it?"

"You better believe it. Today, Bill Hadley, a former councilman. Tomorrow, the honorable Mayor Hadley."

"When you say it like that, it becomes real and scares the hell out of me."

"Don't worry; you'll get over it. Just don't become too cocky for your own good."

"You don't think I would do that, do you?"

"Power can get the best of anybody. But that's a conversation for another time. Go be with your wife. I'll keep the champagne on ice until we leave."

"Thank you for everything, brother."

Bill hugged me. As he left, he wiped tears from his eyes.

That night Liz delivered a six-pound, nine-ounce baby boy they named Christopher Nathaniel Hadley. Linda and I left the hospital at about 2:00 a.m. Bill had won the election, and to our amazement, after he conceded, Rizzo had stopped by the hospital to congratulate Bill and Liz on the birth of their new baby. I felt uneasy while he was there, but his sentiments appeared to be genuine.

———

Bill took to being mayor like a duck to water. After all his worrying and fears, he seemed born for the role. He gave me first choice on what commission I wanted but suggested commissioner of City Health Services, which he thought fit well with my business background. I knew if I took the commissioner position, I would have to get some training in hospital administration to learn the ins and outs of the daily hospital routine.

Another option was to be his chief of staff, working out of city hall as his right-hand man.

The truth was, I was undecided about whether I wanted to work within the system at all. I promised to give him an answer in a couple of weeks.

During that time Linda and I were preparing to become parents as well, with the baby due the following May. I was thrilled for both of us. Our married life so far had been centered around the campaign and the election. Now we needed to decide what path and direction in life we wanted to travel.

We went back to the Virgin Islands to enjoy a second honeymoon and take some much-needed R&R. We were long overdue for a vacation, and I had a lot of thinking and soul-searching to do.

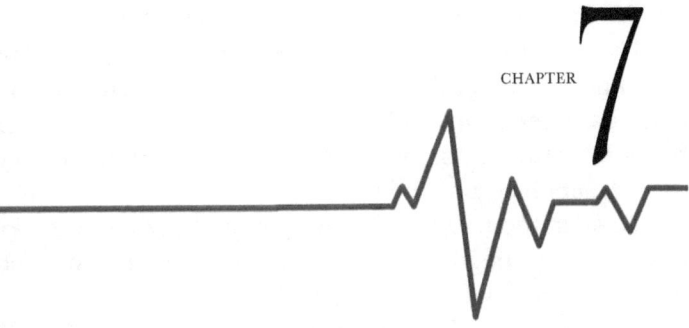

John

Linda and I arrived home from the Virgin Islands thoroughly rested, tanned, and with a plan for the future. I went to see Bill the next day and accepted his gracious offer to become the commissioner of the Department of City Health Services.

"Linda and I discussed it at length and agreed it would be a good start for my career."

"That's perfect." He picked up a folder from his desk and handed it to me. "I took the liberty to look into schools offering a course in hospital management. One of the best is in Atlanta. You would have to go down there for three months for the initial course and then every six months thereafter for a week."

I quickly browsed through the brochure. "My initial reaction is that I don't think Linda will mind too much. She'll be pretty busy with her business and all. Mom will also be around if she needs anything. When will I have to leave?"

"Soon. As in sometime this weekend."

"Christ, you don't give much warning, do you?"

"It's just that the course starts this coming Monday. And I need you to fill the position right away. The current commissioner hasn't collected third-party payments for services rendered for over a year, so the revenue for the department has gone to hell."

"Understood. Do you think you and Liz could make it for dinner tonight? I'll tell Linda before you come, and then the four of us can discuss it."

"Sounds good. I'll give Liz a call."

They arrived around 5:30, and Linda and Liz couldn't break away from one another, sharing stories about Liz's newborn and Linda's impending motherhood. Bill seemed somewhat distant and preoccupied. At one point he barked at Liz for something that was so trivial that I began to wonder about him. It took me by surprise to see him on edge like that. I finally managed a brief moment with Liz to ask what was up.

"Bill's been acting like this since he was elected. I don't know if it's too much for him or what. He's mentioned that a good number of people are approaching him to see if he wants to be on the take."

"Did he mention who these people are, Liz?"

"Not by name. Just that they were already established on the council."

"I would bet a week's salary it's that bastard Adrian Buckley and his gang. He acquired a little power in the council and ran with it. What else did Bill say?"

"As you know, you're damned if you do and damned if you don't. He's torn between his conscience and having an effective policy-moving council. He really wants to be the central force of the city government. Between you and me, it seems the only way for that to happen is to go along with them."

"I don't know, Liz. We all fought awfully hard for an honest election. To go on the take so early is unjustifiable.

I wonder if he isn't running scared before even giving it a chance."

"I know what you're saying, but he needs the backing of the council in order to be an effective mayor. With these dishonest characters on the city council, Bill is powerless. If he doesn't go along with hiring an influential person's long-lost cousin, perhaps even into a nonexistent government position, you know as well as I do that everything Bill attempts to propose will get shot down before it can even be heard by the committee."

I couldn't believe what I was hearing. "It's really unbelievable. Here someone gets elected mayor by the people because they feel he can and will evoke change. He promises them things will turn for the better, and then when he gets into office, he gets hit with all this nonsense. It's no wonder he's feeling the way he does. I wish he had discussed some of this with me before I agreed to become the commissioner of City Health Services."

Bill walked up to join the conversation. "Hey, what are you two in a hot discussion about in the kitchen?"

"We were just discussing some issues I wish you would have told me about. Frankly, you and I've some serious talking to do."

Bill's jaw clenched as he turned toward Liz. "I thought I asked you to wait until I was ready."

"I would have, but Johnny was concerned about your behavior, and I'm not going to lie. And he's right; you two need to talk," she said and walked out.

Bill and I let it go at that and did not talk shop during dinner. But we met the following morning for breakfast and discussed not only his situation but also what exactly my job would entail. I made it clear to him that I wanted full control in any decision-making along with his full support. He gave me his word that City Health Services would have nothing to do with the malignant hierarchy of the council. Taking him at his word, I agreed to move forward.

I spent the week getting organized. I also arranged for Linda to stay with Mom on the weekends. I didn't like the idea of being away at such a crucial time in her pregnancy. She had a family history of miscarriages, so it made me feel better knowing she'd be with Mom on the weekends when she wasn't working.

I hit the ground running in Atlanta, going from the airport to the orientation. There were only eight of us taking this course, with four of my peers coming from the Midwest. Three of us were newly appointed commissioners of a health services department, and the other five were administrators of large city hospitals.

The instructor assured us that the course was designed so we would be able to run any hospital regardless of size and effectively handle its inherent problems. I wondered what variables the instructor might not take into consideration. However, as we got into the program, I began to understand what they meant.

Classes began at 8:00 a.m. each weekday and usually ended about four-thirty in the afternoon. I took more notes than I did in college and high school combined.

It was hard being away from Linda, and I was lonely. I flew home one weekend to see her, but the coursework was too demanding to take weekends off, and I couldn't afford to fall behind. Plus, having to leave after that weekend made me more anxious and feel as though I was missing out. I wanted to be with Linda in case something happened or to just be there to help with the things that used to come so easily to her.

Because the course required all my attention, the weeks ended up going by quickly. Independence Day finally arrived, and as promised, I left with a profound understanding of hospital administration.

When Linda picked me up at the airport, I almost didn't recognize her because her belly had gotten so big. There was no time to relax, though. My new job was waiting. I felt both confident and a little apprehensive. I liked the title Commissioner of Health Services and was delighted to fly on my own after almost a year of being Bill's campaign manager.

That first day, Bill introduced me to Jim Rhodes, who'd been appointed my right-hand man for whatever I needed. He had worked in a hospital since he was fresh out of high school and rose up the ranks. If you needed to know about the goings on within a hospital, Jim was your man. You could see in his eyes that he didn't take to just anyone. He was reserved, and I attributed it to working with two other commissioners over the past six years and seeing hospitals close because of inadequate management.

I had high hopes of proving myself beyond the reputations of others. I just hoped Bill's issues with the city council would not impact running the department as I saw fit.

After meeting with Jim Rhodes, Bill escorted me to the parking lot. There was a new car in a parking space with my name on it. "I hope you like it."

"But I already have a car."

"I know. But this is the commissioner's car, not a personal vehicle. Take a look inside."

On the center console was a phone. "You're kidding me."

Bill grinned. "Besides being a phone, it has a special device that gives you a direct connection with city hall, the hospital, and my office."

"That's a terrific idea. Thank you."

"There's just one more thing. You need to be sworn in today. Why don't you go pick up Linda and bring her back to my office for the ceremony. It's at 5:30."

―

I met Jim in front of the massive administrative building, which was 150 years old and an architectural wonder with myriad design details that would be difficult to reproduce today, like the embossed caduceus etched into the stone above the entrance.

When we walked inside, Jim handed me a long list of meetings I was to attend with individual department heads. He warned me that one of the toughest would be with nursing administration. I laughed.

After the first few meetings, I was astonished at how the hospital could have such a wonderful reputation if what these department heads were telling me was indeed true. For instance, biomedical equipment was a total disaster. The monitoring devices for the intensive care units were twelve years old and outdated, and the engineers barely had the equipment to fix them. The Dietary Department was understaffed and needed updated equipment.

However, my meeting with Mary Gibbons, who had been the director of nursing for seven years, was even more revealing. She arrived exactly on schedule, displaying the presence of a five-star general.

"Mr. West, if I seem like I'm jumping down your throat on your first day in office, I don't mean to. However, I must get through to someone, or you'll not have a functioning hospital because of inadequate staffing and that's a fact. These nurses work their tails off and have not had a raise in three years. We have gotten nowhere with City Hall. It's a wonder that we even have a Nursing Department the way we have been treated."

Before the meeting I had gone over the statistics of the nursing shortage for the past three years. I hadn't known just how bad it was. No wonder Mary was upset.

"Do you have any idea what the nurses do around here?" she asked. "They not only try to give excellent nursing care, but they also have to deal with the pharmacy, dietary, housekeeping, central supply, medical worker departments—you name it, sir.

"They're a special breed of nurses who really care about the welfare of their patients. But they don't receive an ounce of recognition for it. We're so shorthanded nurses feel guilty taking a sick day, so they don't. They're literally getting burned out, so we're losing more and more good people because they're scraped to the marrow."

"And no one has done a thing to improve it?"

"That's correct, Mr. West. I've got the documentation to prove it. We've managed to cover shifts by people doing overtime and by using outside agencies. City Hall has determined we're managing. What they don't see is the back-breaking, difficult work that's involved."

"I would like to review those documents you have and get back to you, if I may."

"Certainly. I'll drop them off at your office. Thank you for listening."

"You're welcome."

After she left, Jim turned to me. "She's tough."

"Is what she's telling me true?"

"I'm afraid so. The nurses are really something here. They work very hard and take a lot of abuse."

"I want you to call all the department heads who are supposed to meet with me at the office and tell them I'll come to their departments. I want to see for myself what's going on. This will enable me to have a first-hand view of what each department has—or does not have—to offer."

At this particular city health services, there were three medical services staffing the in-patient care: Harvard, Tufts, and Boston University. It was from those three medical schools that the hospital's reputation was borne. If it weren't for the competition between them, each wanting to be better than the next and breeding some of the most renowned doctors throughout the country, it would probably not be as well-known. I had heard of this rivalry and wondered why they loved to compete as much as they did and what they actually got out of it.

The meeting with both the medical and surgical directors told a now familiar tale: they were also overworked and underpaid. Interns were putting in roughly seventy hours a week with less than thirty-six hours of sleep. How could they function adequately, and why did their chiefs let this atrocity continue? I was told repeatedly that this was all part of their program for an internship and would likely not change.

The scope of the problems completely overwhelmed me. I couldn't comprehend how all these inadequacies could have gone on year after year.

When I picked Linda up for my official swearing-in ceremony, she could not believe how I was acting. My whole personality had changed since I had left the apartment that morning. I honestly didn't know if I was ready for this massive undertaking to attempt to change years and years of bad habits formed by just about everyone in command at that hospital.

Thank God for Linda. She talked me down, and with her support and reassurance, I would try to do my best.

———

The next day I visited the other two hospitals under the auspices of the Department of City Health Services, which were for the chronically ill and not for acute care. Not only were they better staffed than their sister hospital, they were far more efficiently operated. The difference seemed to be geographic location, with the surrounding communities providing practically all the staffing for those facilities. Because most of the staff lived within five miles of the hospitals, there was much less turnover and more stability.

After my tour of the two chronic care facilities, I felt a ray of hope that City Health Services could incorporate a similar infrastructure. The challenge was being located in the heart of the city. Just like in other big metropolitan areas, there were medical professionals who took a job, stayed six months, and then moved on, using City Health

Services as a stepping stone to a better position. That was a costly proposition because the hospital would take pains to train these people, and just when they got into the swing of the job, they would leave.

Another major part of the crisis was the difficulty in firing any civil servant for negligence on the job. On the rare occasion that happened, it could take years to remove them. It didn't matter to the board how inadequate they were or even if they were a danger to patients. The laws were written to make it virtually impossible to terminate a civil servant. The sternest discipline tended to be transferring them, essentially passing off trouble from one department to another.

After spending the first month gathering information and getting oriented, I got together with Jim and a few advisers to plan out how to purge one of the greatest hospitals that ever existed. It became very clear to me that in order to improve the nursing and house staff situation, we would have to cut back on some of the ancillary help, which was also in desperate straits. But they were the most expendable. The doctors and nurses were my main priorities at the moment because without them the hospital could not function.

My budget was soon handed down by Bill and his advisers. I was grateful they hadn't made any changes to it for the first fiscal year. That allowed me to give some very needed raises while eliminating some of the provisional help.

As soon as we started implementing our plan I began to get threatening phone calls, which Jim assured me was part of the job. I wasn't unfamiliar with this type of phone call after my experience with the campaign, so as long as they remained prank calls I wasn't too concerned.

The long hours spent going over budgets, hearings, and meetings upon meetings meant the time I spent at home was getting shorter and shorter. Linda, as usual, was understanding, but even her patience wasn't boundless. The lack of work-life balance made me even more anxious as the birth of our first child got ever closer.

Six and a half months into the job, word came from City Hall that Bill was putting pressure on them to tighten up the money spent on so-called objects of minimal interest. And apparently the Department of City Health Services was considered an object of minimal interest, so its funding was going to be cut. This meant having to pull teeth for every penny spent. I called Bill immediately.

"What the hell is the meaning of us being included in objects of minimal interest?"

"I'll level with you. The council refused to pass my proposed budget. They claim it was way overboard."

"Was it?"

"I didn't think so, but they claim the city is in debt now—as usual—but this time it's deeper in the red than usual."

"But why pick on something as important as health-care?"

"Politics. The council believes that it's more important to spend money building up the waterfront, which will certainly be more profitable for the city than spending on City Health Services and public works. The hospital was always based on giving free medical care, so it has never made money for the city and is always the first to be cut. They feel the less spent, the better."

The short-sightedness of it infuriated me. "There's nothing more important than the delivery of good health-care."

"I couldn't agree with you more, but my hands are tied. All they envision downtown is the dollar sign."

"I vividly recall that you said you would support my position in your administration."

"I've tried my best, but what can I do? They've tied my hands behind my back. I can submit all kinds of legislation, but you know as well as I that it's up to the support of the council to pass it. I really am sorry. I honestly didn't think that they would put the squeeze so tightly on the Department of City Health Services. All I can ask is that you do the best you can."

"I don't know how I could have been so stupid. I blamed the past administration of this department for the situation the hospital is now in. But now I can see the truth. Sure, they may have skimmed here and there and pocketed a little money for themselves, but it's the people in city hall who deserve the credit for the city's poor healthcare."

Bill sighed. "I don't know if the total blame rests with them, but certainly money has always been an issue."

"And how convenient for you that I wasn't told about any of this before I accepted the job. Had I known, I wouldn't have touched it with a ten-foot pole."

"You have to take my word as a friend that I didn't know all the details. It's all come so fast. The truth is I'm ashamed that the council can dictate the mayor's office. Some of the council members should never have been elected. In my term as mayor, I'm certainly going to see what I can do about it."

My anger cooled because it was a distraction, and I had work to do—purging the hospital. Initially, thirty-two hospital workers were laid off at City Health Services alone. Her sister hospitals were blessed with only fourteen layoffs each because of the longevity and seniority of their workers. I certainly wasn't making any friends.

A week after the layoffs were posted, my secretary was mugged walking to the train station after work. She said two dark-skinned men in their twenties had knocked her down and stolen her pocketbook.

At the time I didn't think it had any connection to the layoffs. But then two days later Jim Rhodes was coming out of a meeting with some of the department heads and was stabbed in the leg by a crazed man yelling about equal rights and layoffs.

He kept screaming, "I'll get you all for taking my job away."

I found out that he was one of the provisional workers let go. It was easy to understand his anger. Thank God there weren't many incidents after that, although the threatening notes continued.

Winter rolled in, and it was one of the worst in memory. We received about forty-two inches of snow before the middle of February. There were a lot of respiratory ailments, with different strains of the flu virus. It was virtually impossible to adequately staff the hospital.

Luckily, we could rely on a few nursing agencies to fill our needs. At first I was told we had no money in the budget for the nursing agencies, but when it hit the editorial page of the newspaper the money couldn't come in fast enough. That was an important lesson learned to remember for the future.

A few months had gone by, and many of the adverse conditions had not improved since I had taken office. I had high hopes of speeding things up; however, I heard from City Hall insiders that Bill was getting tougher all the time.

The job of mayor was certainly changing him, and I guess it would anyone trying to do a good job and putting up with the bullshit he had to face every day. Our friendship was feeling the stress and strain of both our jobs.

The new year came and went. Then it was suddenly spring. I was in a meeting on Tuesday, May 2nd, when Linda called from home saying that her contractions had started and to meet her at Women's Hospital. When I arrived Linda was being whisked into the delivery room. It all happened so fast. It seemed like seconds later when that first beautiful crying sound announced that a baby girl, namely Sara West, had entered the world. What a picture of vitality and so, so beautiful.

As I gazed into the face of this new little being, I remember thinking to myself how tiny her features were and how lucky Linda and I were to share this splendid gift of life. It was the most total and wonderful happening I had ever experienced.

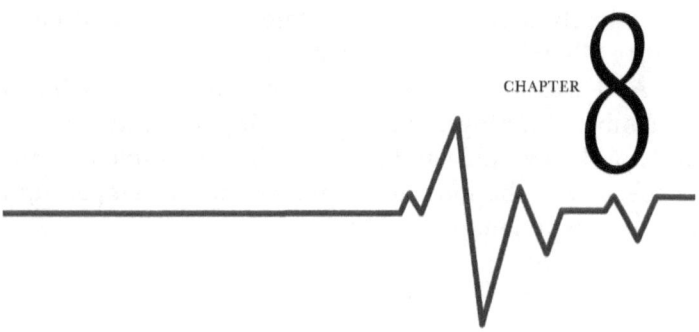

CHAPTER 8

John

A long with the dog days of summer came the new fiscal budget in July. I was feeling more and more resentful toward my job because it kept me from having more time at home with Linda and our new daughter.

Bill was constantly on my back, sending memo after memo telling me I was way over budget. Friendship between us was a thing of the past now; however, I kept in touch with Liz to see how things were going. The pressure of the job had changed him both at work and at home.

I did my best to avoid him. Those times when I couldn't, it would inevitably end in an argument because of the money being spent. I showed him all my facts and figures. They didn't impress him, so we went on a tour of some wards.

I had to laugh. Before we even got through the Intensive Care Unit, Bill got sick and threw the towel in. I had simply forgotten what a weak stomach he possessed, and although he agreed that I was using the money wisely, he said no more. There we were in the back stairwell of the seventh floor, still arguing about money. We wound up back in my office, barely speaking to one another.

He sat across from me scowling, and I thought of how much we had both changed from excited college students to now men in city government. I had heard just a few days ago that in one of the budget meetings discussing the Department of City Health Services that he had said, "Some people will just have to die."

I asked Bill if he really said that.

"Yes, it's true."

"Just what in the hell are you trying to prove? Out of one side of your mouth, you're telling me that you think I'm spending the money wisely, and out the other side, you're saying that people will just have to die because you have to make certain budget cuts. What gives you the right to play God? Answer me that one. This is not you; I want to know what's really going on. Lately we cannot even discuss the weather without bickering."

"Okay, I'm going to give you the facts, and after that, I'll need your complete cooperation in the matter." He paused for a few moments, then continued. "Do you remember a while back when we were discussing the immobility of City Hall and how in order to get anything passed through the council, one had to go along with them rather than fight them?"

"I remember."

"I'm on the take."

I stared at him, my mind frozen. I finally asked, "When did this happen?"

"Not long after I took office. I refused as long as I could, and you have to believe that. Some of the minor legislative pieces I would send down to the council to be approved would get sent back to me without approval for the most idiotic reasoning imaginable. I'm so ashamed of myself. I'm not worthy of this position at all."

"It sounds like the same old story we have been hearing about for years."

"It is, and unless half the councilors are cleaned out, every mayor of this city will have to go through this. They're bloodsuckers."

"Is there any way that we can clean up this whole mess?"

Bill wiped his hand down his face, looking utterly defeated. "Not unless I exposed everyone, including myself."

"Jesus, I just cannot believe all this. How can the people of this city trust anyone?"

"I'm afraid they don't have a choice."

"They did when they elected you. Does Liz know?"

"No."

"I think it would be a good idea if you told her. She's been really worried about you lately."

His eyebrows rose. "You two have been talking?"

"She's afraid because she doesn't know who the hell you are anymore."

"I don't know who I'm anymore. I wanted to be mayor so badly, and now it's all I can do to keep my head above water without sinking into the deep shamefulness I feel right now."

I sighed. I wish you had told me sooner. Although I suspected as much."

"You haven't mentioned your suspicions to anyone, have you?"

"Of course not."

"You'll keep this just between us, won't you? I don't want Linda to know, either. Will you promise me that?"

"Enough already. You know you can trust me."

"I know. I'm just scared."

"I truly feel sorry for you, Bill, but I also feel sorry for myself. Now that I know what is behind the scenes, the damnedest part of all this is that I'm going to have to go along with what you wish. If I weren't sworn in and hadn't already put a tremendous amount of work into this job, I would resign in a minute."

I felt myself getting truly angry. "How the hell am I going to tell people they have to provide maximum healthcare but *'Oh, by the way, you may or may not get your paycheck this week?'* It's going to be impossible for them to accept it. And I'm going to hate myself for knowing what's going on and for going along with it. I wonder if the council would have tried to pull the same shit if Rizzo had become mayor."

"I don't know; they're a powerful group. But my guess is they would not dare push too hard for fear of their own lives."

I kept my word and didn't tell a soul about Bill. How could I? He was so miserable and full of self-loathing and shame that it would totally destroy him if the truth leaked out. I suspected and hoped that he would eventually confide in Liz so she could help and comfort him. I longed for this nightmare to be over.

My own trouble started to materialize when we began to feel the shortage of nurses. Sometimes there would be only one RN along with a nurse's aide to care for twenty-three patients, some of whom were on respirators or other complex machinery.

Nights were even more disastrous. At least twice a week, wards were going uncovered. Patients would die without anyone knowing until the next morning when the day shift arrived. Bill's comment *Some people would have to die* kept going through my head. He was a damn fool to have ever said that. I just hoped not too many would remember, and it was laid to rest.

We had nothing more to offer those nurses to entice them to stay and work for us, and I knew that they would not get another raise for some time to come. The other area hospitals were offering much more attractive salaries and benefits. We were now classified as one of the lowest-paying hospitals in the area.

To my complete surprise, one of the nurses wrote a letter to a daily newspaper about the dangerous conditions within the hospital. The paper published an editorial praising the nurse for coming forward with her information in an attempt to protect her patients. We had to fire her on false premises. It wasn't an easy thing to do, and I was beginning to feel just as dirty as those people at city hall.

All my hopes and dreams of making City Health Services better were vanishing. Jobs would be posted but couldn't be filled because of insufficient funds. But nursing was taking the brunt of it, lacking a strong union to back them up.

The laboratory would only operate until nine p.m. because there was no money for overtime. Some of the wards even had to be shut down for the lack of nurses to take care of the patients. The patients wound up being distributed all over creation. It was a total disgrace, and here I was, the commissioner of City Health Services and not able to do a damn thing about the poor services.

Not a day went by without hearing about a potentially dangerous situation because of low supplies and equipment that was either malfunctioning or not working at all. The reputation of the hospital was slowly but surely going downhill. I heard that one of the council members had gotten sick around the hospital grounds and refused to go to our own emergency ward. Instead he went to a private hospital down the road. I had to laugh. I couldn't help thinking if that sucker was ever admitted here, he probably wouldn't live to talk about it after the staff got through with him.

The lack of funding almost meant I didn't go back to Atlanta every six months to finish my education in hospital administration. Instead I had a front-row seat to what happens when a hospital is dying a slow death. A year and a half into my tenure, our bed capacity throughout the hospital was cut in half from 980 beds to 460.

Then came the disturbing news that the three medical schools that staffed the hospital would be breaking up. City Health Services was being scraped to the marrow, and on a day-to-day basis, people just had the bare essentials to work with.

After a lot of back and forth, University Medical School staffed the hospital with interns and residents and took over both the medical and surgical services.

I couldn't believe that all these changes were taking place. I kept asking myself why in the hell did I ever accept the job, and why did they have to pull this shit during my term as commissioner.

It was a devastating cycle. Many of our patients who had relied on our services before were now drifting away to other hospitals that had better healthcare to offer. Clearly, this sent revenue plummeting. I sent a memo to the heads of the medical and surgical services to attempt to keep the beds filled to capacity regardless of whether the patient didn't need to continue his or her stay in the hospital. This meant that the ICU, which had the largest revenue, was to remain filled at all times.

If we didn't take these drastic steps, the hospital would fall on its feet and close for sure. It would not even get accredited if we couldn't prove that our bed situation was indeed tight. I hated myself for being a part of this. At least the commissioners before me had ample opportunity to improve the situations they were in; they just never gave a damn.

Jim Rhodes got out and quit at the same time the three medical services were departing. Who could blame him? He had seen disasters at City Health Services in the past, but this was too explosive for him. Jim told me that he couldn't stand to be around for the demise of the hospital that he had given so much of his life to. Anyone with an ounce of common sense in their head was getting out before all hell broke loose.

One evening while working late in my office, I decided that it might be a good idea to see what was really going on in the wards by doing a spot check. As I watched the light go from one button to the next on the elevator, I felt my heart begin to race with trepidation. It had been months since I had stepped onto these wards.

It was about 7:30 when I walked out of the elevator onto the third floor of the medical building. On this particular floor, there were only two nurses, one nurse's aide, and an intern on duty during the three to eleven shift. The staff's expressions made their skepticism about my presence clear.

I looked to my immediate right, and there were four elderly women clad in their johnnies with blankets over their legs, sitting almost motionless in their chairs. Braced to their chests were what the nurses told me were posey jackets, which fit snug over the chest and were then tied behind the chair as a protective measure so the patient wouldn't fall out of the chair onto the floor.

One of them was screaming to get back to bed, and another reached out her hand to me and asked if she could kiss me. My heart sank. I was devastated to think that elderly patients existed this way. I leaned over, introduced myself, and gave her the longest hug and kiss I was capable of.

At the other end of the corridor, two elderly female patients in their seventies were screaming at each other and using their metal walkers as armaments in their wrangling. In the midst of this, a very elderly gentleman shuffled by, dropping stool wherever he walked. It was an incredible scene.

Who would believe that this was going on in a supposedly acute medical facility? Part of me felt the urge to run, while another part of me wanted to see what in the hell was going to happen next. Age-old curiosity, I suppose.

As I approached one of the few private rooms down the hall, I heard the rhythmic sounds of air going back and forth at a steady pace. I looked into the room and saw an intubated patient lying motionless in bed. It was a woman, probably in her sixties.

I asked the nurse how long she had been in the hospital, and she said about six weeks. The woman had suffered a cardiac arrest six weeks earlier and had been in a coma ever since. She added that the woman had a Do Not Resuscitate order, or DNR.

"So we're simply waiting for her to die."

"Who and what determines a DNR order?"

"When someone has no or very little brain activity after trauma such as a cardiac arrest, they usually go through a waiting process of days to weeks to determine whether they will ever regain consciousness. In her case, she's not responded neurologically since her cardiac standstill at all."

We were interrupted by the intern on duty. He looked like a kid out of high school. Nevertheless, he was in charge of the floor that night.

"Nancy, can you help me with Mr. Richards in room 304?"

"Sure, just a second." She introduced me to the intern, Bill Garrett, and we shook hands. "I was just trying to explain to Mr. West how a patient is determined DNR. I think that you can probably explain better to him."

"Well, in order to label a patient as a DNR, they need to demonstrate very minimal activity. This ultimately means that the patient has little to no activity in their brain. Sometimes they're very close to brain death but don't fill all the criteria to take them off the respirator."

"What criteria?"

"It's called the Harvard Criteria, which sets out

parameters for irreversible coma: unreceptivity and unresponsiveness, no movement or breathing, no reflexes, and a flat electroencephalogram. Every situation is different. If a patient has in fact been determined to be brain-dead, you need permission from the family to remove the patient from the respirator, after which they usually die right away."

"What if they don't die right away?" I asked.

"Then we just continue to support the patient and comfort him until he dies."

"No disrespect intended, Doctor, but has anyone ever been labeled a DNR who wasn't actually brain-dead?"

"That's a difficult question to answer. It depends on the circumstances and the individual patient. For instance, we had a patient on this ward not too long ago who had a severe respiratory disease and couldn't tolerate being off the ventilator for even five minutes. He was a man in his sixties with a long history of chronic obstructive pulmonary disease, or COPD. Sometimes he would be awake and alert, and other times he would be unresponsive.

"He was on our floor for about three months, and we tried desperately to get him off the respirator but were unsuccessful because of his lung disease. Continued dependence on a respirator for any length of time is detrimental, not only for your lungs but for all bodily functions. The patient also has to be fed either intravenously or through a tube threaded through the nose to the stomach. After extended time on a respirator, most of these patients have a tracheostomy. This is done to try to avoid permanent damage to the trachea from the long tube, such as this patient here has.

"The mortality of this whole arduous process is very high because many of these patients will contract infections that lead to sepsis and die. These patients go through a death worse than hell. Many of those who are coherent will ask us not to resuscitate them because they know they will never recover. But it's a very heavy decision and depends on the individual situation. We try to be as altruistic as humanly possible."

I thanked the intern for taking the time to explain, then made my way home with an empty feeling in my gut. My mind couldn't stop thinking about that poor defenseless woman on the respirator. I wondered how many people in this world were like that. We pass hospitals all the time but never really think about the people inside. Only a small group of healthcare workers knew exactly what was actually transpiring.

I walked into the house after 10:00 p.m. Linda had been a little worried—and a little annoyed—because I usually came home around 7:30.

"What in the world happened? I called your office, and there was no answer. Why were you so late, and why didn't you call? You look so pale."

"I just came from the hospital. I had a bright idea that a spot check would give me better insight. I should have done it a long time ago because it certainly opened my eyes. It's a sad state of affairs. I saw something that's bothering the hell out of me."

"What is it?"

"I came across a woman in a coma who was on a respirator to keep her alive. And she's going to stay that way until the good Lord takes her."

"Why?"

"The intern on duty told me she suffered a cardiac arrest that left her seriously brain damaged. She's not totally brain-dead, so she'll remain on a respirator until she dies, either from infection or some other complication. It bothers me that someone can show no signs of life, be unable to breathe on their own, be brain-dead for all intents and purposes, and not be allowed to die. I think I'll give Sam a call in the morning; maybe he can enlighten me more on the subject."

After we made our way to bed, I lay there staring at the ceiling, wondering: *What if that ever happens to me? Would Linda and my family be able to cope with a decision to remove me from a respirator that was supporting what we know as life?*

I could tell Linda was asleep by her rhythmic breathing. I hesitated to wake her up, but I felt a discussion as important as this should not wait. After nudging her a couple of times, she aroused and sat up with a puzzled expression.

"What's wrong?"

"I know this might sound crazy, Linda, but what if something should ever happen to me, and I wind up on a respirator and brain-dead like that woman I saw tonight?"

She frowned. "Johnny, why are you obsessing about this?"

"Because these situations are real, and if we don't think about them now, then should the occasion arise, decisions could be made without much thought at all," I insisted. "People don't realize how confusing things can be if they don't understand what's going on. I just want you to know that if anything should happen to me where it seems as though I wouldn't be able to function or have much brain activity, I want all artificial means of support stopped. To have a death with dignity would mean more to me than to be stripped of all my controls and suffer needlessly on mechanical devices."

"That's an awful thing to ask of someone you love dearly. I don't know that I could do that."

"And that's why I wanted to discuss this with you so all the decision-making wouldn't be on your shoulders. There's a legal document called a living will where I can stipulate my wishes. I'll give Patrick Carroll down at city hall a call in the morning and find out more about it. If it sounds okay, I'll have him draw up the papers and sign them. That way, the responsibility won't be on you. It's what I want."

"You're really serious about this, aren't you?"

I sighed. "You didn't see that woman. She was so pathetic, lying all alone in a dark room entrapped in her body, unable to move. I can't get her out of my mind."

"I hate thinking about such things."

"I know, honey, but death is inevitable for all of us. I just want to make sure that I don't linger around as a vegetable. This is a way to take care of you and Sara."

"I can see your point, but why the rush?"

"Protection," I said. "I don't want any of my family members having to make a decision that would ultimately change their lives. It's much easier to discuss it now to establish what my desires would be should this happen to me.

"It scares me to think that this woman has no one and is in that room with her body yearning for death. It would be a kindness to disconnect her from the respirator, but nobody can."

Linda took my hand. "You know I'll do anything you wish, within reason. For myself, I'll have to give it some more thought. I hope your mind is more at ease now and you can sleep. Although I don't think I'll be able to."

"Let me show you how to relax."

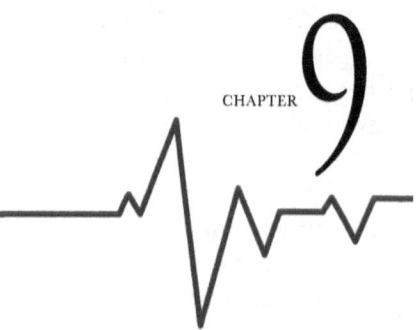

John

During the next few months, the budget crisis continued to worsen. Some of the hospital staff found themselves going without paychecks or being laid off without notice. It was an intolerable situation, and we all suffered.

Even Bill went without a paycheck for a while. Rumors began to circulate around the hospital that it was going to close, and nurses were quitting by the handful. The house officers were picketing City Hall and getting news coverage every chance they got but to no avail.

After many, many meetings with the deputy auditor and Bill, I warned them that the healthcare administered at the hospital was in grave danger, and if they wanted to save the facility, they needed to do something immediately. In one of those meetings, Bill got really upset when I told him to either take care of the problem or close down the hospital.

"What the hell do you expect me to do? There are no answers."

"Someone has got to have the money, Bill. You cannot expect me to continue to run a hospital with no funds."

"We have a $22 million deficit."

"I don't give a damn what you have. There are patients at that hospital going without medical care. I knew you were going to cut some of the funding, but this is ridiculous. I'm sorry, but I cannot in all honesty go on as commissioner of this department if something isn't done so these patients don't suffer. If some capital is not directed toward this hospital, I will quit, and that's a fact."

"I'll try again and see what I can do. Maybe a different approach will work, but no promises, okay?"

"Let me know what's going on and that you're at least trying."

He nodded and then quickly left the room.

I was so damned fed up with the politics of this city that my gut feeling was to get the hell out. However, I also felt that, at the very least, I was a reliable go-between for the hospital against the powerful city machine. The only shining light at the end of the tunnel during this time was that Linda became pregnant again, much to her surprise and mine. Nevertheless, we were elated that Sara would have a little brother or sister. Sara was quite the little charmer and a gentle soul who took to just about everyone.

Mom was thrilled with the news of another grandchild. She was also delighted that Sam was engaged to be married, beaming with joy as only a mother can. Sam asked me to be his best man, and Sara was to be the flower girl. All of these glad tidings were an emotional lifesaver as they kept the problems at work from taking total control over my mind and soul.

I managed to slip away for a week during the budget crisis to go to Sam's wedding in Connecticut, where his bride, Sheila, was from. Of all things, he had married into money. Sheila was the heiress of a pharmaceutical company that her father owned. Meeting her for the first time, one would never know that she came from so much money. She was intelligent, natural in her manner, and radiated warmth and exuberance.

Mom embraced her as a daughter right away, and Sam seemed hopelessly in love. After their honeymoon in Europe, he told me that he was moving his practice to Boston. This made Mom the happiest she had been in a long time. Finally, both of us would be close at hand for her.

The week passed quickly, and when I got back to Boston, Bill and a couple of the deputy commissioners of the hospital were waiting for me when I got off the plane. Bill led us to the terminal's bar, and we sat at a table tucked in the corner.

"So why the reception?" I asked Bill.

"We've got a big problem at the hospital. The interns and the nurses are planning to strike tomorrow morning."

I sat back in my chair. "Jesus, I knew they had reached their limit, but I didn't think that they would do something like this, especially both at the same time."

"That's why I'm here. We know you have a good relationship with these people, and we want you to stop it."

"Stop it? How in the hell do you propose I do that?"

"Talk to them, persuade them that this is no good. We don't need the publicity that this will create."

I looked Bill straight in the eye. "Absolutely not. I'm not going to be the city's gofer."

"What do you mean?"

"Just what I said. I've been busting my ass trying to make you people at City Hall listen about the medical crisis down there, and all I got in return was bullshit, and you know it. Regardless of your situation, I really don't give a damn."

I also understood any work stoppage by healthcare professionals wasn't their choice.

"In case you're not aware, they're striking only because

they want to deliver good healthcare and nothing else. Sure, their weekly paychecks are in trouble, but that's only a minor issue. On a day-to-day basis, there are hardly enough supplies to get through the week. The nursing coverage is beyond crisis intervention, and the doctors are too damned tired after a seventy-hour week to benefit themselves, let alone the patients. And I know this is not news to the people down at City Hall."

"Don't look at me that way."

"Don't expect me to feel sorry for you, Bill. City Hall created this with all their cutbacks. I'm sorry if I make you uncomfortable, but if you want to know my honest opinion, this strike is long overdue. For example, one patient was having chest pain—possibly a heart attack—and when their doctor asked for an EKG machine, it was missing straps to attach the leads to the patient. The nurse explained that when she ordered them, the supplier told her they were on backorder and didn't know when the next shipment would arrive. So they had to improvise and use elastic bands. How would you feel if you were in that bed or someone you loved?

"Another patient had a cardiac arrest, and not only were drugs missing from the crash cart, but when they went to shock the patient, the defibrillator didn't work. The machine had not been inspected by the bioengineering department for weeks. The nurse on the floor had to literally run to another floor to get a defibrillator that worked. The patient died. Whether she'd have died anyway is anyone's guess.

"There are countless situations like this that go on every day. Some are reported and others are not. There are just so many to recount that the staff gets tired of reporting them because nothing is done about it anyway. I won't support the strike, but I'll not have anything to do with stopping it either." I stood up and put on my jacket. "That's my final answer, gentlemen."

I stewed the entire cab ride home and was so angry that I paid for the taxi out of the city's expenses. I tossed and turned all that night. Feeling exhausted and with my nerves on edge, I gave up trying to sleep and arrived at work the following morning very early. Even at 6:45 a.m. the majority of doctors and nurses were lined up in front of the hospital. I had arranged with Mary Gibbons to call in as many agency nurses that we could possibly get from all around to cover the wards, and at the same time I attempted to reroute the patients to different hospitals.

The ironic and most disturbing part of this was that I was allotted extra funding for agency nurses in this crisis situation. Amazing how money comes out of thin air when there's a crisis. My own staff had to abandon their clerical duties and roll up their sleeves to pass around buckets of water for bed baths. It was devastating.

All the attending doctors had to administer direct clinical care to the patients, such as drawing blood and starting intravenous fluids, which they had essentially been away from for years.

Both the patients and the staff were suffering. The agency nurses sent to cover the wards didn't know the patients, and there were some who didn't have any idea how to deal with acute care patients. It was totally out of our hands at this point, and there wasn't anything we could do. Just to have a visible person in white resembling a nurse was cause for thanks.

The first day was bad enough, but going into the second, things got worse with each passing hour. The critical areas, such as the intensive care units, were the priority to be staffed, but when two of our patients were found dead on the same floor, the magnitude of pressure increased exponentially.

News of the deaths somehow leaked out to the press, and City Hall was coming down on me hard. I tried to remain as cool as I could, but they were the ultimate bastards. By the third day, it became so reprehensible that I went out into the streets in front of the administration building, where the nurses and doctors were picketing.

The last straw for me was those patients being found dead, and I asked to speak to one of the broadcast reporters. I felt people had a right to know, even though my job and possibly my life were on the line.

I said, "Patients were needlessly suffering because of insufficient funds to provide day-to-day operations at the hospital, from housekeeping right on up through nursing."

I had taken a stand, and it wasn't with City Hall. In retrospect, it was the only thing to do.

I felt as though a huge weight was lifted from my shoulders as I walked back into the administration building to my office. My comment was broadcasted on the evening news that the strike was indeed necessary for the patient care of the entire hospital.

A few minutes after the segment aired, my secretary buzzed me on the intercom to say Bill was holding.

"I was expecting to hear from you," I told him.

"I don't have to explain why you're fired, then?"

"No. Frankly, I didn't anticipate anything else. Thanks for calling."

I hung up the receiver and sat in my office alone for a few minutes. I buzzed my receptionist and asked that all my calls be held. I needed time to collect my thoughts. What a hell of an ending it was. I felt ambivalent about the whole situation. Through the large window behind my desk, I could see that the crowd had dwindled, and the television crews were gone.

I collected a few of my personal things along with my briefcase and slipped unnoticed out the side door. Feeling somewhat like a failure but at the same time knowing in my heart and soul that I had done the right thing, I left holding my head high, without regret.

The long walk home left me feeling better emotionally

and physically. As I rounded the corner of my street, I could see several TV reporters with cameras in front of my condo building, along with some curious neighbors. I felt a surge of anxiety as I approached. I wanted to run in the opposite direction and avoid them. I wasn't prepared to get bombarded with any more questions. I could only imagine what Linda was thinking.

I took a deep breath and approached my building. At the sound of my footsteps, faces turned in my direction.

Someone called out, "There he is!"

Then everybody began to clap and cheer. I was semi-blinded by camera lights and flashing bulbs as the crowd started chanting my name. I didn't know what the hell was going on, nor why these people were welcoming me like a celebrity.

When I finally got inside, Linda smiled at me and said, "You're the people's champion."

Even more surprising than hearing myself called a hero was seeing Bill sitting on my sofa with a drink in hand.

"What the hell are you doing here?" I asked.

"Just hear me out. First, you're not fired; you're still commissioner of City Health Services. What you did today made you a protector.in the eyes of a lot of people."

I glanced at Linda, and she was all smiles.

"What's this really all about, Bill?"

"The fact is, I've been raked over the coals with all the publicity this strike has caused. In very simplistic terms, you're the victor, and I'm the villain."

"How so?" I asked.

"To make a long story short, the shit hit the fan when you went on television. I heard from the council. They intimated that if I didn't take the blame for not distributing adequate funds for the hospital, they would blow the whistle on where the funds actually went."

"Which was where?"

Bill paused. "This is not easy for me, and I'm ashamed, but the funding went into an escrow to cover raises coming soon for the council, the deputy mayor, commissioners, and so forth."

"I can't believe that you agreed to do that."

"I have practically no control over the council whatsoever. I wish my term were up right now."

"Why don't you resign then?" Linda asked.

"I would if I could be assured that my credibility would remain intact. If I resign now, the council will surely let it leak where the funds went and that I was too weak to take the pressure. Frankly, Johnny, I admire you, and so do most of the dignitaries of the state."

"I find this very difficult to swallow, Bill."

"Difficult as it may seem, it caused a lot of investigating, and there were calls about the two deaths that had occurred during all of this. Because you went public as the commissioner of City Health Services, the hospital will be running smoothly again with adequate funding."

"After I made my announcement, I never dreamed that things would work out this way. I figured I would be fired, and that would be the end of it. What will happen to you now?"

"There will be a couple of investigative procedures that I'll have to deal with. But before I leave this office, my main objective will be to break up that malignant council. Who knows, maybe I'll bare my soul to the community and be a hero, too. The trouble is, who would I find to believe in me? Besides, with my luck, it would backfire right into my face."

"You'll always have us to believe in you, Bill, and don't you forget it."

"Thanks. It means a lot to me after what we've been through together." He drained his drink, then stood. "I must be going now. I need to figure out what strategy to use against these people."

"Thanks for coming by and laying things on the line with me."

"You're welcome."

After Bill left I sat back in my easy chair, thinking of the old days. I wished we all could go back in time to college when life was easier. Bill was a good man caught up in a corrupt system. I didn't want to have any part of the malignant bureaucracy. Both Bill and I had reached our respective breaking points but responded to them in different ways.

For the next two years, things quieted down considerably. The hospital medical staff was much happier with their working conditions, and any request I made to City Hall was usually granted without question.

I was grateful everything seemed to be going extremely well.

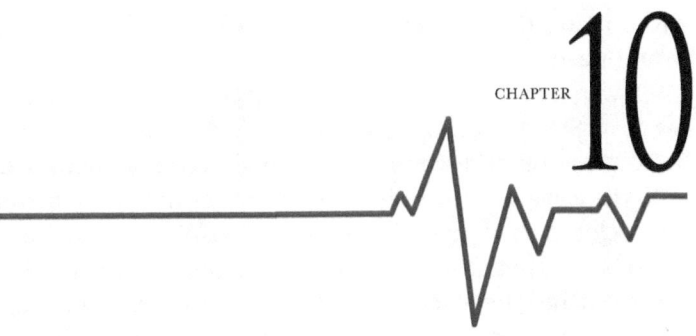

CHAPTER 10

MAC

"**M**ac, has the mayor been notified about the commissioner?"

"I believe the chief resident took care of it."

"Good, good. Try to keep things steady here, will you?"

"I'll try, Brian. If the situation should change, where can I reach you?"

"Just call the operator and have her connect you to the public relations office."

I thanked him while silently wishing that I hadn't been on duty when they brought the commissioner in. If we lost him, they might blame me. It certainly wasn't easy transporting Mr. West to the cardiac care unit. We had to wheel him through long, dark, dismal corridors underneath the hospital in order to reach the medical building.

During transport we attached him to a portable monitor with defibrillator paddles ready to shock him in case anything happened. We weren't taking any unnecessary chances, and believe me, I prayed the whole way. It would have been disastrous trying to code him in the corridor without all the proper medications and personnel we would need.

I watched his heart rhythm like a hawk anticipating his prey. Steadily echoing its contraction, it went beat after beat. My adrenaline level was sky-high as we maneuvered onto the elevator. The only sound heard as the heavy metal doors closed us off from the rest of the hospital was the continuous beeping from the portable monitor reflecting his heartbeat and the whooshing of air from the breathing bag.

The elevator doors opened on the first floor, where a half dozen people were waiting to get on. The respiratory therapist standing at the head of the stretcher near the elevator door held up her hand.

"Sorry, no one can enter. This is an emergency."

A few moments later we arrived at the second floor where the CCU was located. We whisked the stretcher as fast as humanly possible to Room 1, where two CCU nurses were already waiting.

Mary, the charge nurse, asked, "What is the story with Mr. West, Mac?"

"He had some chest pain on the expressway and managed to stop his car. He suffered a cardiac arrest en route to the hospital in the ambulance."

"Give us at least five minutes to get an admission cardiogram and vital signs. What drips is he on?"

"The one in his neck is a keep-open saline with low-dose dopamine infusing into it. The one in his arm is also saline with lidocaine piggybacked into it, infusing at two milligrams per minute."

"Okay. Thanks."

"One other thing. Bob is the admitting intern tonight. Make sure that if you have any questions to get him, okay? I'll be in the back room making a few phone calls. So far, no one has been able to reach his wife and brother. By the way, his brother just happens to be one of the best neurologists around."

"This is going to be awful for them."

"I know."

As they transferred Mr. West to the bed, his hands started twitching.

"Mac, do you see that?" Mary said.

Within moments he was suffering a full-blown seizure.

"Draw up a gram of Dilantin—stat," I told her. "Bob, check his blood pressure while I put in a stat page to neurology."

Once we got the Dilantin into his IV, the seizing eased. Soon after, Sam West walked in. He asked for an update. Although Sam seemed in shock, he gave me some advice about his brother's neurological status. He thought the seizure was caused by insufficient oxygen to his brother's brain from the cardiac arrest.

"Sam, I know you probably want to stay in here throughout all this, but I really don't think it wise. If I need you for anything, I won't hesitate to get you. Do you know where your brother's wife is? Someone has to find out where she is to tell her what's going on. We haven't been able to reach her."

"You mean she's not aware of all this? I have to call my mother and tell her about Johnny. I'll see if Linda is there with the kids."

Tears streamed down his face as he walked out of the CCU. I felt so badly for him. I didn't know if Sam had reached his family, but it seemed some city bigwig was always showing up, getting in the way, and testing my patience.

I finally had to ask the mayor and some of his entourage to leave the unit. They were standing in the middle of the entrance of the CCU, disrupting the whole unit.

Mr. West's heart rhythm had stabilized, but his blood pressure was beginning to drop. That was typical of the type of heart attack he had suffered. The EKG indicated he had sustained enough damage to his heart to go into shock, so we ended up putting him on more vasopressors to maintain his blood pressure. It worked for a little while, but his blood pressure began to drop again.

The director of cardiology, Dr. Cohen, determined we should move Mr. West to the procedure room to perform a catheterization, where a thin tube is inserted through the arm into the right side of the heart to monitor its function.

We also performed numerous other procedures and treatments, trying to improve his circulation and mitigate the damage done to his heart and body. Dr. Cohen had called in two other cardiologists to assist, and everywhere you looked, nurses, doctors, and technicians were scurrying around, focused on tending to Mr. West.

Ordinarily, as the CCU resident, I would be doing the procedures with the help and guidance of the cardiologist on duty. However, in this case it was only the top-notched cardiologists doing any procedure.

But I had other problems and other patients to deal with in the unit. I helped my intern, Bob, with all the scut work, such as drawing blood and completing paperwork.

I was busy in the nurse's station going over another patient's cardiogram who was having chest pain when I heard someone buzzing to enter the unit.

I slid off the stool and ambled down the hall toward the CCU entrance. I glanced through the window and saw a woman, her face etched with pain and anguish. I instinctively knew it was Mrs. West. I wondered how the hell she had gotten down the hall without anyone warning me that she was there. I had left specific instructions that I be notified if she even entered the hospital. I wasn't prepared for this. I cautiously opened the door.

"I'm Linda West. Where's my husband?"

"I'm Doctor James McIntyre. Please come with me, and I'll update you on your husband's condition."

I took her to the waiting area and told her what I knew. "According to the EMT, Mr. West experienced chest pain while he was driving on the expressway and pulled over. Another driver saw he was in distress and called for an ambulance. Your husband was awake and alert when the ambulance arrived, but en route to the hospital, he went into cardiac arrest."

"A heart attack? Oh, my God! Where is he? I want to see him."

She started to stand up, but I put a hand on her arm. "Mrs. West, your husband is alive, but he's in critical condition. I know this is a lot for you to take in, but I also must tell you that he's on a breathing machine."

"A respirator?"

"Yes, along with another device that helps manage the shock he's presently experiencing."

"I can't believe this. He's been in good physical shape all his life. Why did this happen?"

"Unfortunately, we don't know all the answers right now. His brother Sam mentioned that their father suffered from heart problems, and that can run in families."

"Can I see my husband? Please."

"Not right now, Mrs. West. He's undergoing some procedures. I'll let you know when they have him stabilized."

I got Mrs. West a cup of coffee and went back to catching up on paperwork. I knew John West had a snowball's chance in hell of ever coming out of that procedure room alive, and yet I wanted to give her hope.

The buzzer sounded again. This time it was Sam who headed straight for his sister-in-law. They embraced briefly then Linda clutched his arm. I couldn't help but overhear their conversation.

"I cannot believe Johnny is this sick. How could this happen?"

"I know it's scary, but we have to believe he'll pull through this."

"Why him, Sam? He's too young to have a heart attack. And he was fine today. We were supposed to meet for dinner, so your mom came and got the kids. Now he's lying in that room. What are we going to do?"

"We need to get a hold of ourselves and just be there for Johnny."

Linda stared into Sam's eyes. "I can see in your face that you're not telling me everything."

He shook his head. "It's all too early to tell yet."

"To tell what?"

"Whether Johnny suffered any brain damage."

"Brain damage? My God, from what?"

"I was told he had a seizure after he was admitted. That could mean nothing, or it could be related to his heart attack."

Linda sat back and said quietly. "If that's the case, Sam, I know Johnny would never want to survive."

"Like I said, it's much too early to tell. All we can do right now is pray."

"Is your mom coming?"

He nodded. "I called Sheila to go over to Mom's. I'm going to go pick her up. Can I get you anything before I go?"

"When can I go in and see him?"

"Just as soon as they finish the procedures. Let me go see if I can find anything out."

Sam came over to the desk and asked if I could provide an update. I went into the procedure room and talked to Dr. Cohen. Unfortunately, the news was not good. When I came back Linda was also at the desk beside Sam.

"Dr. Cohen says they're having trouble threading the catheter in his arm. So they might want to do a second cut down on his other arm to see if that will work. Dr. Cohen wants to know if you have any objections?"

"No, tell him to do what he thinks best."

"Wait a minute, Sam," Linda said. "Before you start giving permission for anything to be done to Johnny, I want to know what all these procedures mean."

"I'm sorry, Linda. Habit. Of course you have the ultimate authority as next of kin. What another cutdown involves is that they will make another incision in his opposite arm in an attempt to get the catheter to his heart."

"Will it be painful?"

"No, the area where the incision is made is carefully numbed so that he won't feel a thing."

"Okay, they can go ahead. Can I see him just for a minute before they begin the procedure?"

"I'm sure it's okay," I told her. "But it needs to be quick. I must warn you, he's not responsive, and you need to be prepared."

"I know. Thank you very much."

Sam put a hand on her shoulder. "I'm going to call Mom and give her an update."

"Okay, Sam."

"Are you ready, Mrs. West?" I asked.

"Yes."

I took her by the arm, and we walked to the procedure room. I asked her to wait while I alerted Mary that we were coming in. I was relieved when I saw that Mr. West had been covered with a clean white sheet and that some of the blood that had gotten on the floor during the failed catheter attempt had been cleaned.

I brought Mrs. West in, and as we approached the stretcher where he lay, her face became etched with pain. She let out a loud, deep cry, then lay her head on his chest, begging him to come back to her. It was awful. After a few moments I told her we needed to go, but she wouldn't budge. I tried to pry her away from him, but her strength was greater than mine.

"Please, Mrs. West. We need to go so they can finish here. The sooner they do that, the sooner he'll be back in his own room."

"I can't leave him. He looks so helpless. Please let me stay. He's my husband."

"I know, Mrs. West, but we would be only in the way. They won't be much longer." She didn't move. I spoke with as much authority as I could muster.

"Mrs. West. It's important that we let them get on with their work. You need to let them try to help him get better."

Finally convinced, I escorted her back to the waiting room. Her hands shook as she drank some water I got for her. *What does one say at a time like this?* I wondered. It's something you never get used to in this line of work: knowing the patient's chance of survival is next to zero but still trying to provide a glimmer of hope that the person might survive, so they don't completely fall apart. It tears you apart.

Sam returned and sat next to his sister-in-law.

"How's your mom holding up?" she asked.

"Not well. I thought she was going to collapse. I'm just thankful that Sheila was there to comfort her."

"The kids don't know, do they, Sam?"

"No, absolutely not. I told Sheila to tell them Johnny had to work late, you're with him, and that was why they're staying with Grandma overnight. Actually, they were excited to be staying. Miracles have happened before; we just have to pray a little harder."

"Sam, I hope you're right."

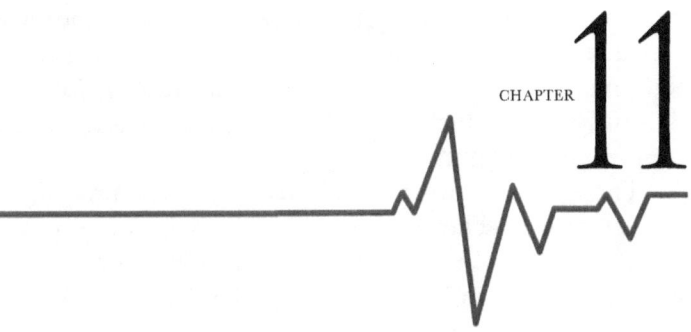

CHAPTER 11

Sam

Dawn was drawing near on Thursday as the last suture was applied to the opening in Johnny's arm. The catheter procedure relieved some of the workload of his injured heart, and his blood pressure was stable.

It had been about twelve hours since Johnny suffered his cardiac arrest, and he continued to remain unresponsive. This wasn't a good sign, although it was still too early to predict the outcome. They let Linda go into the procedure room to be with him while they readied all the machinery for his transfer to his bed.

My heart ached for her as she talked to Johnny with her soft, sweet voice, encouraging him to get better and telling him she loved him. As a physician, I was constantly aware of his prognosis, but as Johnny's brother I refused to believe it.

I accompanied Dr. Cohen along with the technicians, nurses, transportation workers, and respiratory therapist, who all escorted Johnny the short distance back to his CCU bed. It was of vital importance that we guard Johnny's life as if we were Secret Service agents surrounding a president. One false move with this highly sophisticated equipment could mean immediate death for Johnny. Carefully, we inched down the corridor, making a left turn toward bed number one.

There was an otherworldly feeling in the unit. Cool air blew from the air ducts to keep the CCU at a constant temperature for the patients. Periodically a monitoring system would sound an alarm if a patient's heart suddenly did something erratic.

I remembered it was 6:30 a.m., according to the round-faced clock on the wall above the bed, and the CCU had started to come to full life. Overnight the hospital was mostly empty, with hardly a soul walking the corridors. Once in a while you could just barely make out the figure of a nurse checking in on her patients with a flashlight outside the unit. It made me think back to reading about Florence Nightingale with her candle glowing in the dark, checking in on the sick. In this case, the flashlight was used so as not to disturb patients by turning on the room light.

Approaching the bed, a couple of nurses pulled the stretcher alongside the bed in a parallel fashion while the other members of the team placed his life support systems, occasionally bumping against the wall, which had scars of missing paint where it had been scraped by equipment many times before.

With each available person manning a part of Johnny's sheet, we counted aloud to three and lifted him into bed. I stood at the bottom of the bed looking at my brother for a moment, then glanced from the central control monitoring system at the nurse's station to the patients around the unit. I could see some of them were on life support, attached to a machine that provided the continual inhalation and exhalation necessary for life. It reminded me of the sound when I tried scuba diving in the Virgin Islands on my vacation, the constant sucking in of air and exhalation of bubbles going through the vast tubing.

All these sounds and noises could terrify someone who had not the slightest idea of what they meant. As a doctor or nurse, you get used to all the sights and sounds of treatment, making us generally immune to the horror it reflects. Having someone you know and love in the intensive care unit is an entirely different experience. Now the sounds of the machinery seemed foreign and threatening. I felt an unfamiliar vulnerability; I felt scared.

All this was really taking place to my brother, the commissioner of the hospital in which he lay helpless. I knew it would be days, maybe even weeks, before we knew Johnny's prognosis. His face was so pale and placid looking. His six-foot frame looked so minute amid all the highly sophisticated, life-supporting equipment.

The endotracheal tube that extended from his mouth and attached to the respirator was taped securely in place on his face. He had about four lines of intravenous fluid infusing into both arms simultaneously, and with the input of all this fluid came the output of golden urine flowing into a drainage bag clipped to the side of his bed.

One astute young nurse observed that I was trembling as I wiped Johnny's sweat-beaded brow. She came over and comforted me with the reassurance that they would take excellent care of him. I thanked her, and she stood next to me for a few minutes reminiscing about Johnny and the excellent work he did for everyone at the hospital. I nodded and was pleased that she had come over to me.

I sat alone with him for the next few minutes with my hand gripping his, sipping on hot coffee the nurse had brought me, and just staring at him. I kept wishing I could go back in time. I truly felt lost on a different planet. My reverie was broken when I felt a hand on my shoulder. I turned and saw Bill.

"You look exhausted, Sam. Linda fell asleep in her chair. You both have been up all night. Why don't you come downstairs with me and at least have some breakfast?"

"I don't know if I could swallow anything."

"You're both going to need your strength, and it'll do you some good to get out of here for a while. I'm sure you have a beeper, so they can contact you if his condition changes."

I nodded and stood. "I guess you're right. It sounds like a good idea."

I bent over and kissed Johnny, then walked with Bill to wake up Linda. I found it curious how Bill didn't seem to have any reaction to Johnny's situation. I realize each person deals with traumatic events differently, but still, it struck me as rather odd.

When I gently tapped Linda on the shoulder, she woke with a start.

"What is it? Is Johnny all right?"

"Everything's okay," I assured her. "Bill suggested we get something to eat, and I think it would do us both good."

Linda slumped back, looking doubtful. "Maybe one of us should stay in case he wakes up."

"I have my beeper on, so they can reach us if anything changes. Why don't you go see him for a minute? Then we'll all go get something to eat."

She shook her head. "You and Bill go. I want to stay with Johnny. You can just bring me back something?"

I knew I wouldn't change her mind. "Okay. Page me if there's any change."

Bill and I left and hardly said two words until we sat down in the cafeteria.

"How does it look, Sam? Be straight."

"I'm afraid not too good."

"How could he have a heart attack? He was always in the best of health."

"It could be hereditary. Our dad had a bad heart. The bigger issue is that there's a possibility he may have permanent brain damage. Even if he recovers, he might never be the same."

"Jesus, Sam. Is Linda aware?"

"She knows how serious his condition is. What's weird is he told her not that long ago that if he should ever wind up in a situation that would render him totally helpless, he didn't want to be on life support. He wanted her to let him go."

Bill shook his head. "You're kidding?"

"Look, he's seen situations in this hospital that are totally without dignity," I explained. "There are patients all throughout this building that are a hair's breadth from brain death and are just existing. That really made him aware of his own mortality. Linda says he went to see Patrick Carroll, an attorney at city hall, about it. I'm not sure what Patrick told him because Massachusetts doesn't recognize living wills—at least, not yet."

"If there's anything I can do for Johnny or anyone, you have my telephone number. Please don't hesitate to use it."

"Thanks, Bill. I need to call my mom and my wife. Then I better get back to Johnny and see what is going on."

"How's your mom taking it?"

I sighed. "Very badly. I don't know how she'll survive if something happens to Johnny."

"With the hope of God, he'll pull through."

"I hope so, Bill. I hope so."

I tried calling Mom three times, but her line was busy. Frustrated, I went back to the CCU and found Linda crying in the waiting area, her head in her hands. Fear that Johnny was dead caused a surge of adrenaline, leaving my heart racing.

"Linda, what is it? What happened?"

Before she could answer, Mac walked up just as my

beeper went off, followed by the voice message: *Arrest in CCU stat.*

Mac heard the message and grabbed my shoulder. "Sam, it's okay now."

"What in the hell do you mean it's okay now?" I shouted.

"Your brother's heart went into ventricular fibrillation and then flatlined. We had to pump him a couple of times, shocked him, and he came right out of it. The important thing is that he responded promptly. You know as well as I do that with this type of heart attack, an arrest so soon can be terminal. He's strong, and he's going to fight back."

Linda had composed herself. "Can we go in and see him?"

"Sure, Mrs. West, just as soon as the nurses finish what they're doing."

"Thank you. And thank you for all you've done for my husband."

"You're welcome, Mrs. West."

I apologized for yelling at him. Mac waved it off.

"Forget it, Sam. I'll check in with you later."

I nodded and sat beside Linda, trying to comfort her, only there was no comfort to be had. We were both miserable.

"Sam, he's so lifeless in there. No matter how I talked to him or where I touched him, there was no response. When will he wake up?"

"I don't know. But we're getting into the crucial hours now. If he doesn't respond within the next twenty-four to thirty-six hours, I'm afraid the chances of him waking up will be very slim."

"I cannot believe that this is happening, Sam. Twenty-four hours ago we were living our lives, fooling around like children, hitting one another with pillows, and making bets about who would show up late for dinner last night. He said I was chronically late. I said I was on time;

he just always showed up a half hour early. Now, he's lying in there. It's so damn unfair."

I finally broke down and we cried together, leaning on one another for strength. With effort, I composed myself.

"I need to call Mom and tell her what's been happening."

"Do you want me to phone her?"

"No, I need to do this. She'll want to know."

I phoned Mom and updated her on Johnny's condition. Sheila had agreed to watch the kids so Mom could come to the hospital. I told her where to find us, then went back to tell Linda, who seemed more composed when I returned. She had combed her hair and put on some makeup to give her pale cheeks some color. She saw my look of surprise.

"If Johnny wakes up, I don't want to look like a wreck because then he'll worry about me instead of focusing all his energy on getting better."

I admired her hope and courage and began to wonder if the two of us, because of all the physical signs of Johnny's deteriorated condition, had subconsciously lost all hope for him. He wasn't able to respond to us. It was indeed a good sign, Linda putting on makeup. Instead of pitying Johnny and ourselves, we had to take hold and be courageous and fight this battle with optimism that Johnny would pull through. He certainly would not want us morose and despondent without him.

The nurse finally told us we could see Johnny. No matter how brave Linda was trying to be, she looked devastated. He was covered with only a sheet up to his waist because of his 105-degree fever. We suspected that the fever was caused by edema around his brain. The burns on his chest were more evident than before from being shocked by the defibrillator. I explained to Linda the function of the various machines Johnny was hooked up to.

Essentially, all the numbers flashing from the equipment were right on the button, but the reality of the situation was that Johnny remained in a coma.

I left Linda alone to spend some private time with Johnny and went to the nurses' station to look over his chart. I had just finished reading the cardiologist's consultation when I heard Linda calling me. I hurried back to the bed.

"What is it, Linda?"

"Look! His eyes are twitching, and the fingers on his left hand are moving just a tiny bit. It started when I was telling Johnny how much the children and I love him and are praying for him."

I checked his pupils, which were the same as before. I didn't really think that this had anything to do with responding. However, the way his eyes were twitching and deviating in the same direction, I worried it might be some residual seizure activity. But he was fully medicated, so I wondered why it was starting again. I shared my concern with Linda.

"Let me check with the nurses to see if this is the first time this has happened since his second cardiac arrest. Do you want to come with me? I think we'd better be going anyway."

I wanted Linda out of there as quickly as possible for fear that Johnny would start having grand mal seizures again. I didn't think she could bear that, and frankly neither could I.

Linda resisted. "Just let me have a few more minutes. I won't be long."

As I was leaving the room, I could hear her talking to Johnny, telling him that he would get better and that the children loved him. I had to fight back the tears. It didn't matter to her that Johnny was in a coma. She talked to him as naturally as though he were sitting in a chair, awake and alert. I wished I didn't have the medical knowledge I did so I could be just as hopeful as she. For the first time in my life, I resented my own profession.

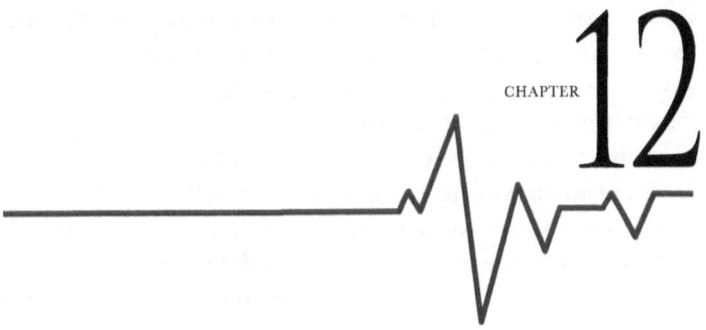

CHAPTER 12

Sam

O n Friday morning Johnny's vital signs were still holding steady, but he remained in a coma. Mom had come on Thursday and cried the whole time she was at Johnny's bedside. Linda finally went home to shower, change clothes, and be with her kids. But she was back Thursday evening and spent the night in a chair next to Johnny's bed. The emotional and physical toll was starting to show. Her usually radiant face looked drawn and pale, and dark circles appeared under her eyes.

I was attempting to hold everyone together and was feeling totally depleted. I knew the longer Johnny stayed in a coma, the more unlikely his chances were for recovery. It kept eating away at me that at some point I would have to tell Mom and Linda that the person they loved would probably never wake up. Amid that uncertainty, Bill had to appoint an acting commissioner to take over for Johnny.

Being the commissioner of the hospital both helped and hindered Johnny. It helped him in the fact that he got the most prominent doctors and the best medical care available, but it hindered him in that he became a threat to some of the nurses taking care of him. Many were afraid that if his condition worsened during their shift, they would be held responsible. It was absurd, so I just regarded it as paranoia and insecurities.

On Friday I arrived at the CCU at about 5:30 p.m. just as the resident was finishing up rounds with the attending physician. I spoke to them both. The neurology attending had been there earlier that day and determined Johnny's prognosis was slim. But nobody had voiced the belief there was no hope that he would ever come out of the coma, nor did I really want to hear it. I was a neurologist; they knew I knew.

By the time I finished discussing Johnny's case with the resident and the attending, it was almost 6:30 p.m. I sat for a moment at his bedside, staring at him as he lay motionless, looking like he was sleeping. Sometimes the only sounds were the constant intake and exhalation of air coming from the respirator.

I was beginning to feel some anger toward him for not waking up. I thought, *How could you do this to me?* and then felt selfish for making it about me. Nothing was in his control. I just needed my brother to come back.

His head and face looked a little better now that some of the swelling had gone down. Both of his eyes were now taped shut to prevent corneal abrasions, which can happen if the eyes open involuntarily and the patient is unable to blink or close them at will.

They had attached leg and arm splints to prevent contractures. They were taken off every four hours, and a physical therapist would exercise his limbs. At 7:00 p.m. a nurse came in and suctioned out the secretions from his lungs, took his vital signs, and turned him. He was fed via a tube that was threaded through the nose to the stomach. A side effect of tube feed for many patients was diarrhea. Being in a coma meant he was also incontinent and had to be cleaned by his caretakers.

I left the room while the nurses got Johnny cleaned up and finished their routine. I felt such emptiness. I got a cup of coffee from the endless pot in the doctors' lounge. As I sat and stared into space, one of the nurses came into the room and approached me.

"I don't want to interrupt, but how are you doing, Dr. West?"

"Call me Sam, please."

She repeated, "Are you okay?"

"No. Have you ever been on the other side looking in?"

She nodded. "I lost my father eight months ago. He had a heart attack, which led to cardiac arrest. By the time he was brought to the emergency room he didn't have a pulse, but they revived him. But his brain had been deprived of oxygen for too long. From the strong and wonderful loving man I knew as my father, he was transformed into a gomer. I was sick."

"I guess you're right. We do have something in common. What's your name?"

"Leslie Adams. What was worse was the way the doctor talked about my father, as if he were a thing, not a person."

"Well, Leslie, maybe we distance ourselves emotionally as a defense mechanism so we can continue to do the job. I became a doctor to help people. But when you have a patient like your father or even Johnny, you feel helpless when there's nothing you can do but wait to see what will happen. Or maybe some of us just become so burned out that we lose empathy toward the patient and family. But if it comes to that, it's time to find a new profession."

"I hate it when I see people dehumanize patients and start calling them by labels: gomer (a patient who does not respond to treatment), DNR, and such. It's a hell of a way to learn what it's all about when you have someone you love lying in bed in that predicament. I wonder when we get off the right track and forget about the feelings and the total essence of the human being beneath all that machinery."

"I wish I knew, Leslie, but it happens all too often."

I had hardly touched my coffee when we were interrupted by one of the other nurses who told me that I could go back into the unit and that Johnny was all set. I thanked Leslie for sharing her feelings with me and slowly walked back to Johnny's room, remembering the neurologist's note.

This patient is not brain-dead by the usual criteria because he has some brain stem reflexes as evidenced by a positive pupillary response, and the ability to take small shallow breaths on his own.

I sat next to Johnny's bed and held his hand. I closed my eyes and almost immediately dozed off. I was awakened by a hand on my shoulder that startled me awake. I turned around and saw it was Linda. I was relieved to see her.

"I didn't mean to make you jump," she apologized.

"It's okay. How is everything?"

"As good as possible, I guess. Your mom is still very upset. I just finished getting the kids to bed, and they're asking so many questions."

"Did you tell them?"

"Not directly, but I'm trying to prepare them." She turned her gaze toward Johnny. "How is he?"

"No change. Why don't you sit here?"

I couldn't imagine what went through Linda's thoughts for herself and the children. I went to get her some coffee, and when I returned, I heard her talking to Johnny again, only this time there was a tightness to her tone. I noticed she had taken the tape off Johnny's eyes.

"What is it, Linda?"

"Look at Johnny's eyes. Have they been following you around like that before?"

"Let me take a look."

"Johnny," I said loudly, "if you can understand me, follow my finger with your eyes."

I went back and forth with my finger, from left to right, then back again. I was astonished. He did it perfectly the first two times but totally missed on the third.

"He understands, doesn't he, Sam?" Linda asked, the hope in her voice almost painful to hear.

"It seems that way."

Tears trickled down her face, and she talked to Johnny with more enthusiasm. I was dumbfounded.

"What made you take the tape off his eyes," I asked.

"I just wanted to see what they looked like."

"Well, good thing you did."

I went out to the nurse's station and asked her to page the chief neurologist on duty. I was afraid to be optimistic because what I had just seen was next to impossible. The data was grim. The overall chance of survival among those who have a cardiac arrest outside of a hospital was just 10 percent. Could Johnny be one of those few survivors?

The phone at the nurse's station rang. The nurse answered and then handed me the receiver.

"It's Dr. Hurst returning your page," she said.

"Hi, Carl, It's Sam West. I wanted to let you know that I think my brother is getting lighter. He's opening his eyes and appears to follow my finger with his eyes on command."

There was a pause. "Are you sure? That seems quite surprising after two days in a coma."

"That's why I called. Can you please come and examine him to double-check."

"I'll be right over as soon as I finish with a patient on the surgical service."

"I appreciate it. Thank you."

When I went back to the bedside, Linda was still talking to Johnny, telling him all that he had missed the past couple of days. I interrupted her monologue to explain why I had asked the neurology attending to come check on Johnny. It was only a few minutes later that Carl arrived.

After I introduced Carl and Linda, he asked, "Is your brother still responding?"

"So far as I can tell."

Linda and I watched quietly as Carl unfastened the bed's guardrail and leaned over so he would be in Johnny's visual field. Carl told Johnny who he was and asked him to blink twice if he understood what he was saying, and Johnny did. Then Carl asked him to follow his finger with his eyes.

Anxious within and calm on the outside, we watched. First to the left and then to the right, up and down. Johnny understood and did it perfectly. But he was blinking more, and his expression was somewhere between a smile and a frown but clearly reflected discomfort.

"When did this all come about, Sam?"

"Just a little while ago. Linda noticed it first. God knows how long this has been going on. They had patches on his eyes for the past couple of days to prevent corneal abrasions. Linda had taken off the patches, and at first it was reflex, but then he responded appropriately."

Carl nodded and then asked Johnny to blink once if he were in any pain. Johnny didn't blink at all. He asked Johnny to move his fingers, first on the right hand and then on the left. Johnny appeared as though he were really concentrating but couldn't move either one.

"That's okay, Mr. West. That will probably come later. You've already made immeasurable improvement by just coming out of the coma you were in the past few days. It'll be hard work trying to communicate, but I'll tell you right now the worst thing that you can do is to get frustrated and give up. You're going to go through hell to get better, but you have to make the effort. Do you understand what I'm saying?"

Johnny blinked twice. Linda stayed with Johnny while Carl and I stepped into the hallway.

Carl rubbed his chin. "This is an incredible improvement, but I would still advise you to take this one step and one day at a time. It's one of the medical phenomena that most bewilders us. And I'm concerned that he's not moving any of his extremities, so let's not get our hopes up too high. This could be a transient situation, as I know you know."

Unfortunately, I did know. "I'm very concerned about my brother's eventual outcome, but I won't lose hope. I can't. Thanks so much, Carl."

"Any time. I'll keep a close eye on him and check in over the next few days to see if there are any new developments."

I thanked him again and went back into Johnny's room. Linda was again talking very softly into Johnny's ear. I thought I could see tears coming from Johnny's eyes. I thought it was best not to disturb such a tender moment and walked back to the nurse's station.

Looking at the wall clock, I realized that I had lost track of time. It was about 9:00 p.m., and I hadn't been in touch with Mom or Sheila all day. I needed to call and fill them in on Johnny's progress rather than wait until I arrived home.

I worried that perhaps we had protected Mom too much and should have let her come to the hospital more often. We worried about her health and the toll Johnny's condition might take on her emotionally as well, but she was probably stronger than all of us put together. I knew I had to be careful not to give her false hope, but on the other hand, I could at least give her reason to have some hope.

Linda and I left Johnny that evening about a quarter after ten to have dinner with Mom and Sheila. As we were approaching Mom's house, the front door opened, and to my complete stupefaction, there to greet us was a ghost from the past: Mary Ellen Brougham.

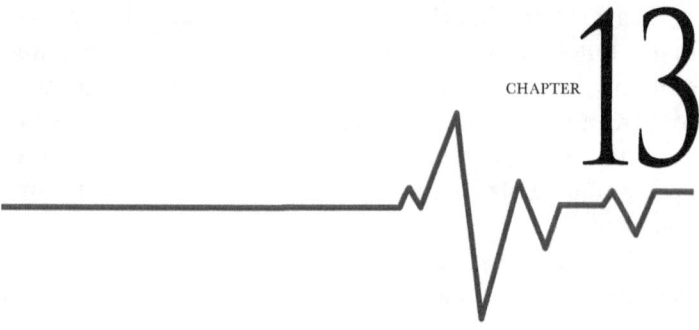

CHAPTER 13

Sam

I hadn't seen Mary Ellen for years, at least not in person. We were all constantly reminded of her in the film section of the newspaper. She explained that by sheer coincidence she was visiting her mother in Boston when she heard about Johnny. I knew that no matter what their differences had been in the past, they continued to remain friends and deeply cared about one another.

She stayed with us for dinner, and we gave her a detailed account of what had happened and his current condition, including his near-miraculous ability to now communicate, even if it was just through blinking.

"Does he recognize you, Sam?" Mary Ellen asked.

"It appears that way, Mary Ellen. For the most part he can answer questions requiring a yes and no answer by the number of times he blinks. But whether he'll continue to regain function or it stops with this, nobody honestly knows. Right now we have to simply wait and see. There is no timetable."

I noticed my Mom looked even paler than she had been since Johnny's heart attack.

"Mom, are you all right?"

She reached out and squeezed my hand. "I think so. It's just when you hear those words said out loud, it makes you feel dead inside."

"I'm sorry, Mom. I just want you to have the truth. That's the only way we can know how to proceed concerning everything."

"I don't know if I should bring this up," Mary Ellen said, "but as you were talking, Sam, it made me think about a conversation Johnny and I had a few months after your father died. He had strong views and opinions about what should happen if he or I ever ended up terminally ill or unable to make our own decisions."

Linda sat forward. "I wonder if he had a premonition that something like this was going to happen," she said, getting everyone's attention. "One night he came home from the hospital after making a spot check on the wards and was unusually upset about a particular woman who was in a coma and on a respirator."

"How long ago was this?" I asked.

"Around the time of the big budget brouhaha."

"So a couple of years ago."

"Right. It was something I really didn't want to talk about, but he insisted; he was practically distraught. Johnny made it clear to me that if he should ever end up like that woman, he wanted everything disconnected and to die with dignity. He even went so far as to draw up a living will with a lawyer down at city hall. But then he didn't bring it up again. And neither did I because I disliked discussing the subject," Linda said, looking guilt-stricken.

Mom shook her head and sighed. "You know, that's my Johnny, always thinking of someone else and how to ease their suffering. He hasn't changed much, has he, Mary Ellen?"

"Not from the sound of it."

I looked at my watch. "It's late, and we all need some

sleep, but let me just explain about the living will. While Johnny might have wanted one drawn up, to my knowledge, a living will isn't recognized in Massachusetts—at least not yet. That could be why Johnny didn't bring it up again, Linda. The point of a living will is to keep the family from having to make the decision to pull the plug or whether or not to stop resuscitation efforts. It prevents people from ending up like the woman Johnny saw that night, being kept alive by artificial means on a respirator. I think what we need to focus on is the remarkable progress he's made and to fight alongside him for his recovery."

"Do you think it would be okay for me to visit him later in the day tomorrow?" Mary Ellen asked.

"I've no objections," Linda said.

I told Mary Ellen, "I think he would be thrilled to see you."

"I *know* he would be," Mom added.

Mary Ellen gave us a grateful smile, and we all finally called it a night.

—

The next morning I got to the hospital early to do an unofficial neurological exam to see for myself if there was any change to Johnny's condition. There wasn't. Before heading home the night before, I made plans to meet Mom and Linda in the cafeteria at 10:30, so we could all go to Johnny's room together.

The cafeteria was full, mostly with hospital personnel taking a mid-morning break. I spotted Mom and Linda sitting at the far end of the cafeteria. Walking up I saw Mom was anxious and noticed she was tightly clutching her rosary in one hand. They stood when I reached the table, and we headed to the CCU.

With all the grace and courage she could muster, Mom approached Johnny's bedside. He appeared asleep. Through her tears she gently kissed and caressed his hand

and ran her fingers through his thick, black hair. She looked at the machines he was hooked up to and asked me what they were for. As I was explaining, Johnny roused and saw Mom for the first time. He just stared at her as she gently talked to him.

"Johnny, it's Mom. I hope you can understand and see me. Oh, how I've missed you. I've all the faith in the world that you'll get better and come home soon. Sam says you've already made remarkable progress. I love you so much."

Mom placed her head next to Johnny's, still whispering words of love and encouragement. His eyes remained opened and flowed with tears.

Linda and I left Mom to have time with Johnny and went back to the cafeteria for some coffee. When we returned an hour later, it was quickly apparent the visit had done them both good. Mom's spirits were much improved. Johnny was asleep, his expression the most peaceful I'd seen since he'd been at the hospital. We chose not to disturb him. Mom and Linda were going back home to the children. I thought I would return to my office. I had some patients that I wanted to check in on. Linda had my pager if anything happened.

It would be good to take a break from the hospital. Maybe it would give me more objectivity about Johnny's case. Sometimes when you're consumed in a situation, objectivity can be easily lost.

I saw my last patient at quarter to five and managed to cross town to the hospital in twenty minutes. My first stop was at the nurse's station to get an update on Johnny's progress. Not too much had changed except that the nurse felt that he was sleeping more than usual and was opening his eyes less frequently. This wasn't surprising. Once he'd opened his eyes yesterday, he'd barely closed them.

For the past day and a half, he'd been running a low-grade fever of 100 degrees. That was also not surprising, considering the extent of the damage to his heart. Being on a respirator didn't help matters either. As I was glancing through Johnny's medication list to see if he was on any antibiotics that would superimpose an infection, Leslie Adams approached me. She was in charge on the three to eleven shift.

"Hi, Leslie. How do you think he's doing?"

"Holding his own and sleeping most of the time, except for now. A woman is in there talking to him at this moment. She said that you told her it would be all right for her to visit. She looks very familiar."

"That's Johnny's good friend, Mary Ellen Brougham."

"The actress?"

"Yes."

"I knew she looked familiar to me. She's been in a lot of movies."

"Yeah, she's made it big. Mary Ellen lives in LA now, but she was born and raised here. She and Johnny were very close growing up. They were high school sweethearts, and I always assumed they'd get married one day. But they went their separate ways after college."

"You could tell there's a very close bond between them just by the way she talked to him and held his hand."

"Did he respond to her?"

"I'm not sure, but his eyes were open."

"I think I'll go over and see how Johnny's doing before I go home. I promised Linda and my mother that I'd report if there were any changes, good or bad. I'm afraid everyone is getting their hopes too high for a complete recovery."

"How about you?"

"I'm trying to be realistic, but I haven't given up hope either."

I walked down the hall to Johnny's room. Mary Ellen was sitting quietly beside him, holding his hand. I gave her a silent wave and leaned over my brother.

"Johnny, how are you feeling?" I asked.

He just stared at me and closed his eyes.

I looked at Mary Ellen. "Is he responding any differently than what I described last night?"

"The only thing I noticed is he seems to have a twitch on the left side of his mouth that comes and goes."

"It may be just reflex, but I'm going to give him a short neurological exam."

"Do you mind if I stay?"

"No, not at all. This won't take very long."

Mary Ellen watched as I poked and prodded Johnny's eyes, mouth, arms, and legs for the next few minutes. When finished, I looked at Mary Ellen.

"What is it, Sam?"

"I didn't see any twitching, but there's more lethargy today compared to yesterday. I'm going to go ask the nurse if he got any additional medication today."

"I'll wait with him until you get back, then I need to leave. I have an audition in LA tomorrow, so I have an 11:00 p.m. flight out tonight."

"Okay, I won't be but a minute."

I walked over to the nurses' station. "Leslie, do you know if Johnny received any additional medication today?"

"I don't think so, Sam, but let me check." Leslie flipped through his medication sheets. She shook her head.

"No, nothing additional. Same as yesterday."

"He seems more lethargic this evening."

"Maybe it was an emotional day and wore him out."

"You're probably right," I said, hoping that was indeed the reason.

I stopped just before entering Johnny's room to glance through his bedside chart, where his vital signs and daily weights were recorded, when I overheard Mary Ellen telling Johnny not to worry, that she'd take care of everything.

As I entered the room, Johnny seemed more awake

and appeared as though he was absorbing every word Mary Ellen was saying to him. When she saw me, she hugged and kissed him and said she'd be back soon.

She hugged me and handed me a piece of paper. "Here's my number. If there's any change, will you please call me?"

"Of course."

"Take care of him, Sam. No matter what happened in the past, I'll always love your brother."

"I know that. And Johnny knows it, too."

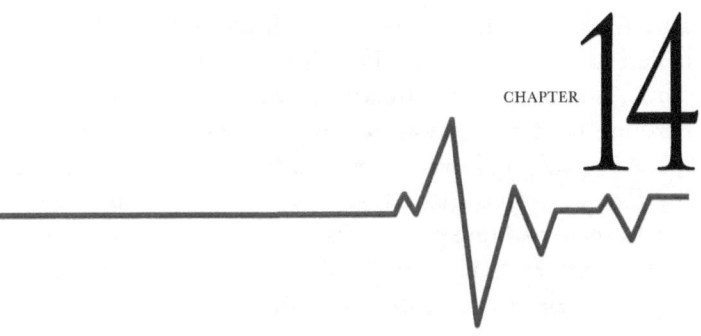

CHAPTER 14

Sam

A day and a half later, Johnny's fever spiked to 103.6°, and he was put on antibiotics. Although his blood pressure and heart rate remained stable in the following days, and the twitching Mary Ellen had mentioned wasn't always evident, his lethargy had markedly increased and seemed to consume him. For reasons nobody could explain, Johnny was becoming almost totally unresponsive, and his eyes were either wide open or closed most of the time.

Another CAT scan revealed no further extension of his anoxic brain damage. Nor had he suffered a massive cerebral bleed, which would cause the unresponsiveness. He was beginning to slip into the abyss, and we all knew it. He had gone through so much, and right now his body couldn't take much more.

Linda shortened her visits to half an hour each day as the disappointment I had warned her about was beginning to take an emotional toll.

Seven days into his hospital stay, the hospital called me at midnight. Johnny's blood pressure was dropping, and he was experiencing an unusually fast heart rate called tachycardia. Even though I knew such a call might come, it still took my breath away and sent a bolt of fear through my body that almost made my knees buckle.

After calling Linda, I dressed as fast as I could, thinking that he would die before I even reached the hospital, but Johnny had one plus on his side. His body was young and strong. He had responded immediately to the medications to elevate his blood pressure, but in turn the drug severely compromised his kidneys. Essentially, Johnny was now experiencing shock. His EKG had shown that he had extended the original heart attack of seven days prior, meaning he'd had another heart attack.

During the short time he had responded to us, he never once indicated he was experiencing chest pain. The enigma was finally unfolding. Sometime within the past couple of days, with or without his knowledge of chest pain, he was beginning to compromise his heart by this extension.

We were all so concerned about his response to us—or the lack of it—that no one concerned themselves with the fact that it could be his original problem that brought him to the hospital in the first place, his heart, which was causing his increased somnolence. He had also developed a staph infection in his arm where the catheter had been placed. So his lethargy and unresponsiveness were from a lack of cardiac output and an infection.

Mom and Linda were up all night at the hospital. They could only get a glimpse of Johnny during the brief intervals that the medical team wasn't working on him. Finally, at 5:00 a.m. his blood pressure stabilized without the aid of a massive amount of medication. He was comatose but alive.

I went to tell Mom and Linda the good news and inform them they could see Johnny as soon as the nurses cleaned him up a bit. Mom was wide awake and busily knitting, and Linda had her head resting on the arm of the chair.

Mom looked up at me. "He's all right?"

"For the moment."

The tension released from her face. "Oh, thank God." She stopped knitting and got up to get Linda and me some coffee.

As I sat down and paused for a few moments, I studied Mom and wondered where she got her inner strength from. Here I was, the son and doctor trying to protect her from all of this horror, and she was the one who possessed the most fortitude.

The coffee soothed my parched mouth. I held onto that Styrofoam cup with my two hands wrapped around it so that the soothing heat warmed my palms. I sipped the coffee, inhaling the aromatic steam. Since Johnny's heart attack, I'd become hyper-aware of the simple things we usually take for granted and how much they contribute to the beauty of life.

It was almost 6:00 a.m. when the night nurse came in and told us that we could see Johnny. His room had even more machinery in it, and their various hums, buzzes, and beeps didn't allow for much tranquility. Besides the heart monitor and respirator, he was also now hooked up to three IV medicine dispensers. It was as though he were on remote control.

I thought back to Johnny's conversations with Mary Ellen and Linda. *Johnny would never want this,* I thought. *How can we let this go on?*

His head was beginning to swell from the infusion of fluid needed to maintain his blood pressure. His kidneys were not handling the increased fluids, so they had no other place to go except the tissues.

Linda held his hand, staring into his face as if looking beyond into a different world. Mom cradled his head in her hand in a comforting gesture. She talked to him as if he were awake and conversing back.

"We are the luckiest sons in the world to have such a mother," I said under my breath to Johnny.

Along with the extra fluid Johnny was retaining, he was also beginning to show the physical signs of being bedridden for an extended period of time, including bed sores, tape burns from intravenous sites, and thinning skin that was more prone to tear and become infected.

With exhaustion and depression overpowering us, we began our journey home at 7:00 a.m. to get some rest. There wasn't much else we could do for Johnny at this point, but we needed to take care of ourselves, and that meant getting some sleep. Before leaving, I asked the charge nurse, Leslie, to contact us if anything should come up.

She looked at me with compassion, but her tone was professional. "With Johnny's failing heart and poor condition, does his wife want him resuscitated again if need be?"

I glanced over at Mom and Linda, then said, "Yes. As far as we're all concerned, right now we want everything done for Johnny. Be sure to call if there's any change."

As we left Johnny behind and walked toward the elevator, the feeling of emptiness was overwhelming. We waited in silence. The elevator had just arrived when I heard the PA system.

Code Three, CCU, stat. Code Three, CCU, stat.

My face went hot, and I whirled around and ran back to Johnny's room, thinking, *This could be it, this could be it.* When I saw the crash cart outside his room, reality struck like lightning. *Oh God, I'm not ready for this.*

I rushed into his room, and my heart sank. He had cardiac arrested and was surrounded by a team of doctors and nurses. His face was grayish blue, his lips pale. I thought I might vomit. Leslie hurried over to me.

"What happened? He seemed stable when we left."

"His heart rate plummeted, then it just stopped."

I heard her voice, but I didn't know if it all was sinking in.

She pushed me back into the hall. "I'll come get you when we know what's happening."

"I'm not leaving."

"You can't be in here right now."

The resident running the arrest told her it was okay as long as I stayed quiet and out of the way. So I just watched and kept out of it.

I stood there helplessly watching the medical choreography required to resuscitate.

"Let's give him more cardiac epi."

"Okay, stop pumping."

"We have fine V-fib."

"Everyone back; okay, shock him."

Johnny's body jerked upward and uncontrollably twitched for a few seconds after receiving 400-watt joules applied to his chest.

Leslie came over and whispered to me that she was going out to the lounge to sit with Mom and Linda. I thanked her and my eyes started to fill.

In the meantime Johnny received sodium bicarbonate to correct the acidosis that occurs during an arrest. His head would bob up and down like a lifeless mannequin each time his chest was being pumped.

"Let's give him another bicarb and more epinephrine and calcium," shouted the resident.

After the fourth defibrillation and more than ten minutes of procedures and chest compressions, he had a heart rhythm and was sustaining blood pressure. But he looked so pathetically grotesque that I almost wished they had not gotten a heartbeat back. His once youthful, attractive body was now a distortion of the human being who was once John West. His neck and head were filled with so much fluid that his facial features were totally disfigured. Smack in the middle of his chest was a large black bruise from the pumping, along with friction burns from the defibrillating.

With his eyelids so swollen, it was difficult to assess his pupils, which were probably fully dilated from the medication he had received. His whole upper torso was exposed, with numerous syringes tossed helter-skelter on the bed. Some of them were empty of medication, and some were half filled with his blood that by this time had clotted.

It was a scenario for a horror movie. I had been a witness to many arrests before, but never of anyone so close to me. My head began to pound as the nurses began to clean up the area, which was cluttered with a massive number of needles and syringes on the floor.

What the hell are we doing to you? I thought again and wondered if he felt any of this. Staring blankly at Johnny, these questions kept going through my head.

It was so inconceivable this had happened to my brother. I felt a fury ignite within me. Here he was, the commissioner of the Department of City Health Services, questionably alive, covered in needle punctures.

No one should ever have to go through that kind of torment to stay alive. It was so damn inhumane. I had to ask myself: *Why aren't we letting go when it's so obvious that Johnny is gone? This cannot continue.*

I walked toward Mom and Linda, who were staring into space, fighting the crushing dread they felt. One glance at Mom's face and I fell to the floor on my knees and cried like a baby. To me Johnny was already gone.

Mom knew it without me having to say a word. She bent down and put her arms around me. Even though part of me felt so dead inside, I felt her strength flow into me, and I was able to gain control of myself.

Linda thought by my initial reaction that Johnny was dead. I knew it was actually worse than that. His heart was in such a state that his life expectancy from that alone was reduced by half. Beyond that, he'd suffered definite brain damage, but to what extent was impossible to tell. His kidneys had also virtually shut down.

After I explained what had happened, we were now faced with a moral and ethical decision nobody wanted to face. We could either put Johnny through more resuscitative measures so that we would know that everything possible was being done for him, or we could do nothing and let nature take its course. He would be a DNR.

We waited another twenty-four hours, and Johnny remained the same. On the tenth day, we had a conference with Johnny's cardiologist and neurologist. Somehow pushing our grief aside, we all managed to put the facts into perspective and together arrived at the most humane decision. With much pain and difficulty, we agreed that Johnny was not to be resuscitated. He would only receive comfort measures as he went from this world into the next, salvaging his dignity.

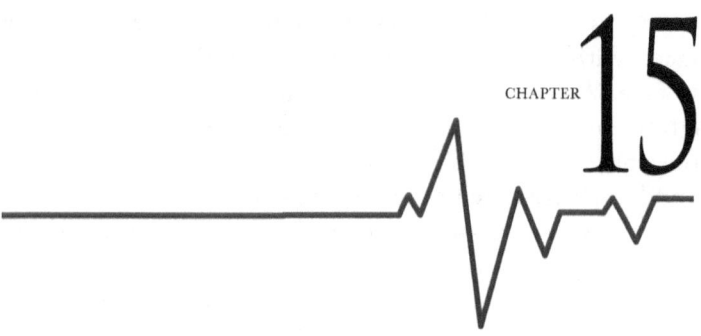

15

Sam

I n a considerate gesture, the medical team kept Johnny in the CCU for the next couple of days. Of course, he was the commissioner of the hospital, so it was only proper to extend him and his family that courtesy.

Johnny's tremors and twitching had ceased, so his body was completely motionless now. His chest was the only moving part, rhythmically moving up and down as the respirator provided breathing. Without it, he would die. One intravenous line remained for a sedative, antibiotic, or whatever. And the tube in his nose remained for nutrition because no one knows if an unconscious patient feels hunger. All these were comfort measures as well as prolonging life to some extent.

We were all drained emotionally and physically. The loneliness of watching and waiting for someone to die was agonizing. It was hard not to anticipate death being a relief and release.

Linda started spending less time at the hospital, feeling the need to stay close to her children. They needed to be her top priority. She explained to them to the best of her ability what had happened to their father, but of course they didn't really comprehend the situation. One night I was at Linda's for dinner when Sara asked when her Daddy was coming home.

I thought Linda was going to burst into tears. I took Sara into the kitchen and talked with her about how Johnny's heart wasn't strong. When I finished, she looked straight at me.

"I know Daddy will be all right. He's going to go to heaven."

She then put her arms around me, hugged me for a couple of seconds, and ran off playing as if nothing had happened.

Children are sometimes smarter than we give them credit for. It made me wonder if children sometimes see things from a much better perspective than adults do. On the other hand, I also pondered how much they block out of their minds that comes back to eat away at them later in life.

After Johnny's heart attack, we all blocked out the possibility he wouldn't make it. Even after the second one, we never discussed Johnny's death and what we would do if he should die. And when he responded to us, we chose to cling to hope as a way to avoid having hard conversations. Now we had to accept the inevitable.

On his thirteenth day in the hospital, Johnny was transferred from the CCU to the third floor and labeled DNR. His electroencephalogram showed his brain was not functioning properly, but it was not totally flat either. Therefore he was not brain-dead. Also, he could sustain taking shallow breaths on his own, so the respirator could not be disconnected. Since the EEG ruled out brain death, he had to be kept as he was.

Being on a general medical floor rather than in the CCU, which is geared to save lives, made us acutely aware that there wasn't more to be done for him.

Reality set in like a thunderbolt. Although invasive procedures and extraordinary life-prolonging measures for Johnny had ceased three days earlier in the CCU, it had somehow been reassuring just knowing he was there. We were able to sleep nights. Now that he was transferred to another floor to die with dignity, we couldn't help wondering what kind of care he would receive.

The floor nurses were just as competent as the ones in the CCU; that wasn't our worry. It was just that we all knew this was the grand finale, and it was overwhelmingly difficult to cope with.

The third floor housed thirty-three other patients besides Johnny, but he was in a private room with only the company of his respirator. He would no longer be cared for on a one-to-one basis as he had been in the CCU. The patient care was divided between three or four nurses per shift. If for some reason there weren't going to be enough nurses for a shift, a private duty nurse would be called in to take care of Johnny.

The single rooms on the floor were much larger than the individual cubicles in the CCU but were rundown. Johnny's had dim lighting, paint-chipped walls, a cracked linoleum floor, an old bedside table with its door broken off, one straight-back wooden chair, and an over-the-bed table. To the left of the doorway was a sink. All in all, it reminded me of a prison cell, including the presence of roaches.

It certainly wasn't the most aesthetic room to have one's own death, but for Johnny, who had worked so hard for this hospital, it would be exactly what he would want. He was never one for fanfare.

There was a suction apparatus and oxygen attachments on the wall behind Johnny's head. The sound of the respirator was more pronounced in this more isolated room, plus there was no competition now from other machinery.

Lying in the bed in the room where he would eventually die, Johnny looked like he was sleeping. His facial swelling had gone down, so he looked more like himself, which made it hard. I kept wishing it was a dream and that I would wake up and the nightmare would be over.

The nurses came into Johnny's room every three to four hours to suction, turn, and give Johnny his tube feeding. But as a DNR, the viable patients on the floor were the priority. Johnny would not take precedence.

As word got around that Johnny was terminal, many of his friends backed away—even Bill and Liz, his most trusted friends through the years. To my astonishment they had only visited Johnny twice in the CCU. It made me wonder if I'd been guilty of similar neglect in the past.

As a physician and a human being, did I sometimes unconsciously abandon a patient when there was no hope of recovering? People don't like to face what makes them uncomfortable, and most people avoid thinking too much about their inevitable demise. Maybe that's why it's a rare few who will stick by through thick and thin.

It brought to mind an article I'd once read by Jim Castelli called "Death with Dignity."

> In the past, when doctors couldn't do as much for their patients, they felt obliged to offer comfort, at least. Nowadays, when doctors can apply a number of sophisticated treatments, personal attention has suffered. Oliver Wendall Holmes reportedly said to his doctor, 'Don't just do something, stand there.' That, in essence, is the modern challenge in providing a good death ... not to abandon the dying entirely to medical technology, but to connect death with dignity, to life with dignity.

That was essentially what Johnny wanted. However, as fate sometimes deals its cards, this wasn't the case. He'd gone through a roaring hell fighting for his life and was now connected to machinery with very little dignity. Abandonment was already in progress, with friends and family alike drifting further and further away. Some couldn't be at Johnny's bedside because they couldn't tolerate to see him so helpless. For others, well, when there's no hope of recovery, why bother?

As a physician, it all hit home. I could remember going on rounds and not even stopping in the room of a DNR patient. We all took the situation as a matter of fact. What was the use? We didn't have to examine the patient because he was going to die anyway.

I thought back to these feelings—or lack of—as I watched Johnny lying motionless in bed. *Where in the hell has modern medicine gone today?* I wondered. *We can try to help a patient live with all our technology, but when do we draw the line and help a human being die with dignity— without being called a murderer?*

While reflecting on these thoughts, it occurred to me that I should call Mary Ellen to tell her about the change in Johnny's condition. I knew she'd want to know. Johnny would want her to know.

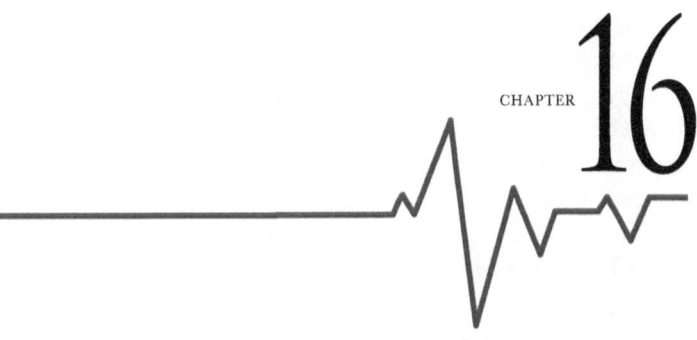

CHAPTER 16

John

I felt entombed within my own flesh.

Why me, damn it? I loved life so much. I had two beautiful children and a lovely wife. In the moments when it felt like my heart had exploded, theirs were the faces I saw before everything went black. *Why was I being punished? It's not fair.*

I thought back to those moments when I'd come out of this endless tunnel of darkness and could see my family. It was so wonderful and so fleeting. Then the abyss engulfed me again.

It had been years since I saw Mary Ellen. She could see in my eyes what I wanted. I was glad someone caught on—certainly Sam didn't.

I used to be able to move my head slightly. Now, I couldn't even open my eyes. I wondered if anyone knew I could think, that I was still here encased within this inoperative, paralytic body? I wished I could scream out and tell everyone *I'm here! I'm here!*

Maybe if they knew I was a thinking individual, they would have visited me more often. Mom and Sam remained very faithful, but I didn't hear Linda as much. My old friends, Bill and Liz, I hadn't heard once.

When I was awake in the intensive care unit, I used to have the same nurse almost every day. Now there were so many different ones at different times that it was difficult to keep track. From what I could gather when they talked, no one wants to have a comatose patient day after day. I guess I couldn't blame them.

I thanked God for the nurses who came in every four hours or so. At least they were consistent. My routine didn't change much. In the early morning, I got a cold bath. It was the rare individual who at least cared that the water was warm. Only certain parts of my body were capable of feeling the water, and when it was cold, I spasmed all over. It felt like hydrophobia. What a dreadful feeling. Sometimes I wished they would let me lay in my own sweat; at least I'd be warmer.

I got turned and my linen changed. Just like a young infant, I was incontinent. It continued to amaze me that hardly anyone talked to me while they were in this room doing their duties, sometimes for a good long while.

Antoinette used to talk to me, but she hadn't been around for some time now. The only conversation I heard was when two nurses came into my room at a time, and they talked to one another. If they only knew I existed in this unconsciousness, they would be horrified and bribe me not to talk if I was suddenly able to do so. Oh well, what they didn't know won't hurt them.

I wished I could awaken and let them know what goes on here in the unconscious. Then again, I wondered if it would matter anyway.

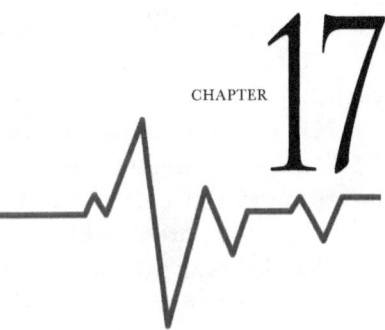

The Nurses

"Come on; let's get Mr. West done up quick. I'm behind and have to give out my 9:00 a.m. meds."

"You know, I don't mind taking care of patients like him."

"In what way?"

"Well, comatose patients don't give you any trouble. You do them up for the day, and that's it. I can't stand patients that pick at things."

"Yeah, I know what you mean, Jill. If you get behind with the other patients and don't get back to someone like Mr. West, well, he's better off."

"Do you want me to ambu him while you suction him?"

"Sure."

"He coughs a little while you suction him."

Jesus, they ram that catheter down my trachea as if it were a steel drainpipe.

"Oh-oh. I'm suctioning up a small amount of blood. I must have traumatized him a little."

"Well, I wouldn't worry about it. At least he can't feel it."

That's bullshit, you two. One day you may have the chance to find out.

"Do you want to change his whole bed?"

"I guess we might as well as long as we are here. There's no telling when we'll get back to him, and we might as well make him look presentable."

"You know, it's difficult to believe that he was once the commissioner of this hospital."

"I know. It's hard to believe, but apparently he was good."

"Listen, why don't we give him a tube feeding before we change his whole bed. That way if he goes, we won't have to change it a second time. Makes sense, right?"

"Good thinking. He'll probably tolerate a double tube feeding, actually."

"Did you hear about the patient who was admitted last night?"

"No, who was it?"

"Some guy came in about 3:00 a.m. reeking of alcohol and complaining of abdominal pain. He's been in numerous times with pancreatitis, so they felt obliged to admit him. They dropped a nasogastric tube and gave him Demerol for the pain. Apparently, all he wanted was the drugs. After two shots, he pulled out his own tube and high-tailed it out of the hospital. The night float was bullshit. He was working him up most of the night when he bolted. What a guy."

"I'll say."

"Is that tube feeding almost in?"

"Just about. Okay, all set."

"I'll turn him to you first since he's way over on your side of the bed."

"Okay."

"Do you think he'll need a plastic sheet where he's been having diarrhea from the tube feedings?"

"No, I don't think so. If he does start to have a massive amount of diarrhea, we'll just insert a rectal tube. I'll load up his bed with bed pads anyway."

"Good idea."

"Over to you he goes. Do you have him?"

"Yeah, I think so. He's a sort of tall fella, isn't he?"

"He's at least six feet, and you wouldn't think he would weigh so much after being in this state as long as he has. Are you ready to turn him back to me?"

I'm just like a piece of meat being tossed back and forth. Who in the hell ever thought I would be in this predicament? Any modesty I ever possessed has vanished. I'm always exposed.

"Just a second. I want to put a pull sheet under him to make it easier rolling him back and forth. Okay, here you go. Oh, shit."

"What is it?"

"He just had explosive diarrhea all over the clean sheets."

"What a pain. I'll never get my 9:00 a.m. meds out on time."

"Just relax a minute. I'll go and get some more linen, and while I'm at it, I'll get an order from Steve for a rectal tube. Do you know what room he was last in?"

"I think he's right across the hall in Mr. Sweeney's room."

———

"Listen, Steve, we need you to write an order for a rectal tube for Mr. West."

"Why?"

"He's having a massive amount of liquid diarrhea."

"I'll write for it, but only for twenty-four hours. You know this place. Once those damn things go in, people just forget to take them out. In the meantime, I'll also write for some tincture of opium to be added to his tube feedings."

"That will be great. Thanks a lot."

"Anytime."

———

"It's about time you got back here. The stench is killing me."

"Sorry. Here's new linen and a rectal tube."

"All right, let's put it in before we change his bed again."

"Right."

"How much air do we put in the balloon?"

"Some people put in thirty cc's, but I think that's too much. Just put in 10 cc's, and we'll hope for the best."

"Look, it's already working. Look. The diarrhea is so serous it's coming right through the tube into the bag."

"We'll leave him be for a while and check him in a few hours."

"Okay, but don't ask me to help you with another thing until all my 9:00 a.m. meds are given out."

"All right."

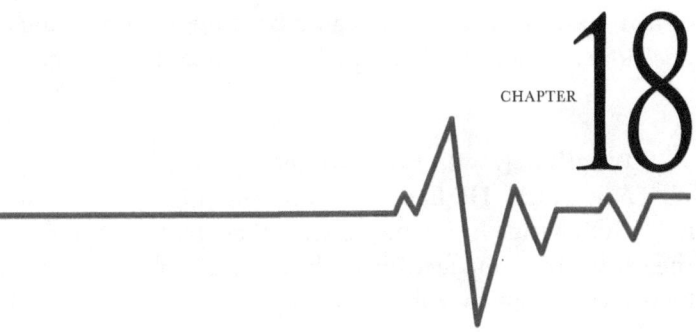

CHAPTER 18

John

A new addition to my already complicated ensemble: a rectal tube in my anus. How disgustingly inhumane.

I wondered what they would think of next. I had a tube to collect every excretory process known to mankind. I felt uncontrollably barbarized in the most modern of times. Lucky for me that for the most part, I couldn't feel most of their invasions. The only pain I felt was in my unconscious mind. No one on the outside could hear, see, feel, or insert a tube into that. Thank God!

Just before I drifted into that black abyss of darkness called sleep, I heard some commotion around the foot of my bed. I recognized the voice of Steve Morgan, who was the intern in charge of my case now that I was out of the CCU. I also heard Dr. John Phillips, who was an acquaintance from my time as commissioner. He was probably the attending physician on the ward. He was a nice enough fella to work with on a professional basis, but I wasn't impressed with some of his teachings. As a matter of fact, I almost had him released because of some radical decisions. For my sake, I hope he'd calmed down some.

—

"What's new with Mr. West today, Morgan?"

"Not much. He had an uneventful night with absolutely no change in his neuro status. He had a lot of diarrhea from the tube feedings. The nurses took care of that by inserting a rectal tube."

"Is that quite all?"

"Yes, Dr. Phillips."

"Has his code status been written?"

"Yes, sir. It's in the doctor's orders that he's a DNR."

"I've spoken to his brother, Sam West, who is a neurologist. The family's conclusion is that they don't want anything done that will prolong the inevitable. It's a damn pity. Such a good man with so much to contribute to life. Oh well, let's get on with the next case."

—

So that's why no one had fussed over me too much since I left the CCU. I was a DNR. I was placed here to die. A nobody with no place to go but six feet into the ground. Like the woman I saw that night in the hospital.

I thought I heard the nurses say that I was a DNR, but I didn't know if I had heard them correctly. At one point, I heard Morgan loud and clear.

As a DNR, why didn't anyone protect my own right to die? I had to wait until some infectious process took over to do me in. Where's the God-damned justice in life itself? Where was Sam? Where were Linda and Mom? The children? Where was everyone?

—

I was awakened by a different nurse taking my temperature. I was startled when I heard her press the nurse call buzzer. A few moments later footsteps walked quickly into the room.

"Susan, will you repeat Mr. West's temperature with a glass rectal thermometer and see what you get? I took it with an electric rectal probe and got 105.6 degrees."

"Sure."

I recognized the second nurse's voice. It was the first time I'd heard her name. Although I couldn't envision her, Susan had a sweet voice and a warm manner. Occasionally while she was in the room administering her duties, she'd speak to me. Things like: *It's such a beautiful day outside today, Mr. West.* It was a treat because it was done so rarely.

Susan told the other nurse. "I get 106.2 degrees."

I was aware of feeling hot and sweaty. A temperature that high couldn't be good.

"I'm going to page Steve Morgan," said the first nurse. "I would think he would want to treat this. In the meantime, Mr. West has a Tylenol order for a temperature of greater than 101.5. Would you put some down his tube?"

"Sure."

I felt so relaxed and comforted having Susan near me, talking to me as if she saw me as a whole human being. The other nurse returned, breathing heavily.

"Steve answered his page and said for us to put him on the cooling blanket."

If my memory served me correctly, she was probably out of breath from pushing the cooling blanket into my room. Back and forth I went across the bed as they got the cooling blanket and sheets put in place. After a while, they finally had me settled and ready to go.

"Okay, why don't we start him off at 96.8 Fahrenheit and check him in an hour? That will be about five p.m. We don't want him to get too cold."

Thank God for Susan's compassion. I was grateful for someone mentioning the time, even though I had nowhere to go. I never had any idea what time it was, what day it was, what year or month.

It was sometime later when the doctors came into the room on their rounds again. If I got used to this routine enough, I could probably begin to tell what time of day it was.

The nurses had just finished taking my temperature again when they arrived. However, this time I had difficulty hearing them because they weren't next to my bed. They must have been just inside the entrance to my room.

I could make out that Steve was updating a new intern about my case.

"The only new development with Mr. West is that he spiked to 106.2° this afternoon. He got some Tylenol down his tube, and he's on the ice blanket now. Susan, what's his temp now?"

"It's down to 103.8°."

"That's good, thanks."

A familiar voice joined the conversation.

"Hi, Dr. Morgan, glad I caught you. How's Johnny?"

"About the same, Sam. He's had some diarrhea and a high fever."

"How high?"

"It spiked at 106.2° rectally. We gave him some Tylenol, and he's on the ice blanket. Right now, his temp has come down to 103.8°."

"That's good. Do you have a source?"

"Not really. It could be his thalamus, or he could have an infection. Whatever, we're obviously not going to culture it."

"I know, it's just habit to ask."

"I understand."

"We'll treat everything symptomatically and give him all the comfort measures possible. I'm going off duty now. Dr. Cohen will be here if you need anything. And if your brother's status changes, we will let the family know."

"Thank you both."

Except for the ever-constant swoosh of air going back and forth from the respirator, silence filled the room for what seemed an eternity. But I could feel Sam's presence even though he remained quiet for a long period of time. The only senses left for me were hearing and a minimal amount of feeling throughout my body, which came and went.

My vision was now totally gone, which left me with only the memory of faces and expressions. I remembered seeing Mary Ellen visiting me. That seemed as if it were in another galaxy, in another life perhaps. My brain played games with time and space. It was as though you're trying to grasp for something and could never quite touch it. You're in a space where there's no gravitational pull.

As I tried to sort out my thoughts, I heard Sam speak.

"Oh, Johnny. I wish you could hear and understand me. If only I could trade places with you. The kids need you so much. You deserve a full and wonderful life. This isn't right, even if God is all-knowing and powerful up there."

He started to sob and apologized for any wrongdoing he might have done as a kid. He was asking forgiveness for something he never did. I love that kid brother of mine.

Eventually, the sound of crying stopped, and he spoke softly.

"I know the only way to help you now is to release you from this trap. I wish I was brave enough, but what a life-changing decision that would be for me."

I knew what he meant, but of all people I didn't want him to be responsible for my inevitable destiny. He'd worked too long and hard to be a doctor, and it would destroy his career, which would devastate his life. I would gladly bide my time rather than put him at risk.

Sam stayed with me for a long time. He was my only visitor from the family that day.

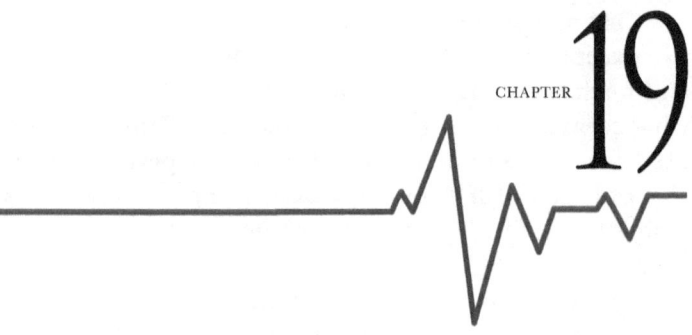

CHAPTER 19

The Nurses

"Susan, we're pretty much caught up with the meds, so while we have a chance, why don't we do Mr. West up for the evening?"

"Thank God it's eight o'clock already."

"Only three more hours in this hellhole tonight."

The nurses were in my room for another check and routine change, feeding and suctioning me as they went along. For the most part, they were truly discontent with their profession. I tried as commissioner to help with their increase in wages because I knew that they never got paid enough for what they had to put up with.

But there were many other factors besides wages that contributed to their discontent. I suppose tending to people like me, a DNR who was incontinent and unable to do anything for himself, among other depressing aspects of the job, made it difficult on a day-to-day basis to remain happy in their profession. I remembered how distressed I was after making a spot check on the medical wards when we had all the trouble with staffing, and all I was doing was passing through.

"Do you want to get the basin and fill it with water for his bath? It looks as though he's stooled around the rectal tube."

"Sure, and I'll get a bunch of bed pads too."

"Great."

I could hear the running of water in the distance with the clashing sound of it hitting the basin as it gushed from the faucet.

"Let's do the routine before we clean him up. If we do it together, we can whip him up faster. We'll suction him out, tube feed him, and check his temperature afterward when we roll him over to clear him."

"Okay."

If there's one sound that you begin to hate, it's the sound of suctioning. It's reminiscent of the final flow of water passing from the sink into the drain, the slurping and gurgling vibrations of water being sucked up by the drain. My adrenaline kicked up every time I heard the whir and whistle of it. I occasionally coughed in a spasm when they would suction me, and that was awful.

I was frightened at the thought of it, knowing at the same time that I needed it. It was a love-hate relationship. You loathe it because it takes your breath away, but after it's all done, you're grateful because it's a wonderful relief when all those secretions are removed. It's like a breath of fresh air.

"Do you have plans for the weekend?"

"David and I have a wedding to go to Saturday, and then I'm covering Mary's shift on Sunday. She's going to a huge family reunion upcountry."

"That was good of you to do that on your weekend off. There aren't too many nurses on this floor who will do that, you know."

"Yeah, I know."

"So Susan, have you heard the latest?"

"About what?"

"Chris is dating the night float. What's his name?"

"Kevin Walsh."

"Yeah, that's him."

"Well, I hope she knows what she's in for."

"From what I understand, old Kevin has the reputation of being the stud of the year."

"She must be aware of that, don't you think?"

"Well, if she doesn't, she's either dumb, naive, or both. One of the nurses in the CCU overheard a conversation with him telling the resident, and I quote, *I'm out to lay as many nurses as I can while I'm here, and man, it's so easy.* They all laughed as they went through his list of conquests, who shall remain nameless."

"What a bunch of assholes. Someone should fill her in on what's going on."

"You're right; someone should."

"You know, they must cull a stud in every group of interns that comes through this place. There is always one. I guess you just have to be around here for a while to know what's going on."

"Yeah, it sure looks that way."

"I'll roll him to you first, Kathy."

"Okay. He didn't have as many secretions this time suctioning him as he's had in the past."

"I know. Over to you he goes. He leaked a little around the rectal tube, but otherwise it looks as though it's working okay."

"That's a plus in our favor."

"And his temp is down to 102.6°."

"Great, let's give him some more Tylenol down the tube and keep him on the ice blanket. They can recheck it around midnight."

"Sounds good to me."

"Have you ever seen Mr. West's brother, Sam?" Susan asked.

"No."

"He's quite handsome and looks a lot like John. He's also a neurologist."

"You're kidding?"

"No. He's got quite a good reputation too."

"Why then is he letting all this go on? Why don't they just let him go?"

"I think everyone wishes it were that easy. But according to the EEG he's not legally or medically brain-dead. So we can't interfere. We just have to wait until the good Lord takes him."

"That could be months—even years. I hope nobody I love is ever in this situation."

"I know. We're done here. Let's go down and do up crotchety old man Mr. Wallace. He's probably been sitting in diarrhea since supper time."

So that's why Sam had not done anything to help me out. The damn EEG still showed signs of activity. I don't think he would have hesitated otherwise. He must have felt awful. If anyone could have communicated with me and know what I wished, they wouldn't have any ambiguity about disconnecting this damn machine.

I wished Mom was there to talk to me. She might have the guts to do it. It's such an awesome responsibility. That's why I made out that stupid living will. What good did it do me? My lawyer, Patrick Carroll, did warn me, but so what? What good was I to anyone like this? What happened to humanity and the essential element of comfort?

CHAPTER 20

John

The night was uneventful, as most nights were. Conversation between the nurses during these hours was generally minimal. The graveyard shift hours, between 11:00 p.m. to 7:00 a.m., were the most peaceful and the loneliest. I could always tell the beginning of the day by the nurses coming in in the morning, alive with conversation and whipping me up, as they called it, faster than any of the other two shifts. The day shift nurses' conversations were usually juicier than other shifts too.

Before I knew it, the crowd of doctors was in my room on rounds again; same time, same place, only another day, 24 hours later.

"Anything new on Mr. West overnight?" Dr. Phillips asked an intern.

"Not that I know of, Dr. Phillips."

"What do you mean you don't know? Don't you check in on your patients throughout the night?"

I heard someone flipping pages of what I assumed to be my chart. "Yes, sir, but I didn't see any reason to check on Mr. West. If there was something going on, the nurses would have paged me."

"I'm not going to go into this right now, Dr. Walsh, but I'll say this. Just because a person is labeled DNR, it doesn't mean that we don't care for them. They're still a patient who deserves our respect and full care."

I heard Steve say hello to everyone and apologize for being late. The night float and Dr. Phillips continued their rounds. Jonathan Cohen stayed behind to fill Steve in on my condition.

"First of all, Mr. West's fever is down, but there's nothing else new."

"What was going on as I came on rounds? It looked as though Kevin was about to kill someone."

"Well, that someone was Phillips the Attending. He let Kevin have it for not checking on Mr. West all night long."

"Was he busy with other patients?"

"He didn't say. I meant to warn him that Phillips and Mr. West knew one another before all this happened."

"He should know that, Jonathan. Anyway, thanks for covering for me."

"Anytime."

It seemed like hours had passed before the nurses came back into the room again, so I had a lot of time to think. I wondered why I hadn't heard from Bill. We were such good friends once.

I thanked God for my mother and Sam; they never failed me. Linda . . . why did she come so infrequently? Maybe the night float was right. Why should anyone bother with me when my destiny is my demise? Would I do the same?

I'd never forget how upsetting it was to see that woman in a coma. The thought of seeing someone you loved in that state—the state I was currently in—without hope for recovery would be devastating.

I had no right to judge anyone.

I wished people knew that my mind was alive and that I could have communicated in an abstract manner. I wouldn't advise it as a steady diet, but each human being should have a taste of deep unconsciousness, for they would have more respect for a person in a coma. It's very disturbing to one's psyche to be tossed back and forth in the bed like a piece of meat. All the controls that existed before were gone.

It was as though I didn't belong in my own body. Not only was I incontinent, but I was also aware of drooling. The nurses would bitch about that because I would drool on the bed as soon as they put on fresh linen. It was like being an infant—including being fed. Not by a bottle, which might provide some comfort, but through a tube. However, there was one main way I differed from a baby: the love and care and sense of being so very much wanted.

Love, the main ingredient for life. It's what it's all about, isn't it? Who took the time just to hold my hand or hold me close so I wouldn't be afraid? Is it so much to ask? I may not have felt anything, but I certainly would know that someone cared, and I would have felt safe. I need that so desperately to pass from this life to the next. It would have given me the courage and strength I needed to go to my death with the dignity I deserved.

I was startled from my thoughts by the ventilator alarm sounding. I'd been gagging and coughing on my secretions much more lately, which caused the ventilator to pop off and disconnect. Within seconds a nurse rushed into my room. After a moment she called out to the other nurse that I was all right. My coughing had dislodged the ventilator. After some suctioning, she put me back on the ventilator, and I was breathing easily again.

Funny. I must not have missed those breaths for that short time. I was just relieved to have the coughing spasm stop. When the nurse left, I tried to cough again but was unable to produce enough pressure to pop myself off the ventilator. But then again, unless someone turned the alarm off, popping myself off the ventilator would be fruitless.

After what seemed like just minutes later, two of the nurses were back in the room to whip me up. They started with the usual suctioning, tube feeding, etc. Susan's voice was familiar to me, but the other nurse's voice I couldn't make out.

"How long were you away?" asked Susan.

"For about three months."

"Where did you spend all that time?"

"Nebraska. I worked out there for two and a half months."

"What the hell made you go out there?"

"Well, I had some friends out there, and I desperately needed a break from this place, so I quit."

"How did you like it?"

"Nice place to visit, but I wouldn't want to live there."

"What were the people like?"

"They were nice enough, but they go at a much slower pace than we do. It drove me a little crazy. That's why I'm back here now."

"Do you have any plans?"

"I might go back to school and study law. Anything but nursing. More and more nurses I talk to are unhappy with their jobs. I love nursing. I wish we were appreciated more and had more support from the administration. Mr. West was our hero. He gave us so much support, and now he lies in an unconscious state. He was our voice when we had none. Who is our voice now? It would be so satisfying to see Mr. West pull through and go home to his family. If only he could respond and let us know what he wants. In times like this you wonder about your own final exit. Why do some people suffer so much before they die? It's so unfair."

"I can't believe that I'm in a profession that doesn't get recognized for what it really is or does. For the most part, it's a thankless job, and people will scrape you to the marrow at times until you're so burned out that you want to switch professions.

"How is Mr. West doing?"

"His fever is almost back to normal," Susan reported.

"Good. Have any of you seen Chris?"

"I think she's in the nurses' station getting her coat to go home."

"Thanks."

After Kevin's footsteps grew fainter, the second nurse asked, "How long have Chris and Kevin been dating?"

"I'm not sure. I think she's only dated him a few times."

"He's got some reputation following him."

"I know."

"Does Chris have any idea?"

"I'm not sure, but if she doesn't, I'm sure she'll find out for herself whether the stories are true or not. Besides, I find it difficult to believe about Kevin. He just doesn't strike me as the type."

"One never knows what lurks behind that virginal white uniform, now does one?"

All the trials and tribulations of life, I thought to myself as I lay helplessly, drifting in an almost fluid-like state. At least where I was going, there would be no bickering or uncertainty. Peace and serenity would finally be mine. I longed for that day to come.

Momentarily, I thought I heard footsteps approaching my bed and felt a slight rush of air go by my face. I could have sworn I was kissed by someone.

"Johnny, it's Linda. I don't know if you can hear me or not, but I want to ask for your forgiveness. I've been afraid to come to the hospital. It's no excuse Johnny, but I really have been terrified to come. It was hard accepting that you were never coming home to the children and me again. I secluded myself with them. But because of them I found the strength to face this and be with you. I only hope you'll find it in your heart to overlook my fears of losing you. Our lives have changed so much. We've been turned upside down. The children keep asking for you. They send their love to you and want desperately to come in and see you.

"I'm going to talk to Sam this afternoon to ask him what he thinks about them coming to see you. I know if it were up to you, you would not want them to remember you this way. On the other hand, they know something is wrong and have got to hold onto something tangible."

Again, silence filled the room with only the ventilator sounding. Minutes later, Linda was sobbing. I desperately wished for it to be all over. It was as though I was already dead and buried in people's minds, with both Linda and Sam asking forgiveness and saying goodbyes. I longed for the strength to be able to reach the ventilator and turn it off, so that would be the end. But I couldn't move.

I suppose for them to talk to me this way while my body was still warm and alive helped them go through the inevitable grieving process, but it was agonizing for me. It was all well and good if they wanted to do this at the funeral, but at that time, it was tearing me apart. Then I heard another familiar voice that soothed me.

"Linda, are you all right?"

"Mary Ellen! Am I ever glad to see you."

"Sam called me a few days ago and explained what's happened, but I wasn't able to get away until today. I'm still in shock. When I left, he seemed as though he was improving so much. How are you holding up?"

"Barely. I'm glad you're here."

"Does he respond at all?"

"No, nothing. He can't even hear us, but we talk to him just the same. Although I haven't been here to see

Johnny for several days. I just couldn't take it anymore, so I stayed with the children."

"You were at Johnny's side through the most crucial period. The children need you more than ever now that Johnny won't be coming home."

"Oh, I try to keep telling myself that, but it eats away at me that I didn't want to see him like this knowing there's no hope of him ever recovering."

"Are they totally sure of that?"

"Yes. His most recent cardiac arrest left him virtually—but not completely—brain-dead. And he's able to take small breaths off the ventilator on his own. That's why they won't take him off the machine and let him die with dignity. By law we're going to have to wait until nature takes over. Or he gets an infection, which they won't treat."

"This was the very thing he feared."

"And yet, some part of me still doesn't want to let him go. But all we can do is pray that God will be good and take him."

"How is Johnny's mother doing?"

"Surviving is about all. She looks more worn and tired as the weeks go by. If it weren't for the children, I don't know what she'd do. I know she'll be glad to see you."

"Do you think we could all get together for dinner tonight? You can come over to my mom's. It would do you all good to get out of the house."

"That sounds like a good idea. I'll call Sam to see if he and Sheila are free. I better be running along. I'll call you tonight."

"Okay. I'm going to stay a few more minutes."

"See you at dinner then."

Linda's footsteps walked away, and Mary Ellen was quiet for several moments.

"Johnny, I wish I could snap my fingers and make this whole horrible ordeal disappear for you. I'm sorry I took so long getting back here. The studio wanted me for a

Western. God, I haven't ridden a horse since we were kids down on Cape Cod. Those were fun times. We were so innocent and young, not a care in the world. First love and so, so beautifully innocent. I still sometimes wonder what would have happened if we had married. Knowing you, we'd probably have six kids by now."

Her laughter turned into tears. It was so painful. I wanted to reach out to her.

"Despite what's happened, there's something about you that seems so tranquil, so peaceful."

"Excuse me, ma'am. I'm sorry for interrupting your visit, but we just received Mr. West's blood cultures back from the laboratory, and we have to place him on strict isolation precautions."

"Why?"

"He had a high fever the other day, and they drew some blood cultures to see if he had an infection. He's tested positive for a staph infection. He'll have to go on wound and skin precautions, which means that anyone visiting with him will have to wear a gown, gloves, and a mask at all times for their own protection. I'm sorry, but it's for the other patients' protection as well as yours."

"How long will this go on?"

"Probably not for long. Because he's DNR we won't be giving him antibiotics."

"Well, I guess I need to be going then. I'll be back tomorrow."

A moment later I heard Susan say, "Okay, let's get this over with. Put the masks and gloves with the clean linen outside the room, and we'll put the precaution bags in here for soiled linen and trash."

"It's going to be more difficult coming in here now, having to gown up and glove for each changing."

"I know."

After they left, the room was quiet for a long time. Now that I was on precautions, I probably wouldn't hear people as often. Too bad. Even though I couldn't see them anyway, it was comforting to hear their voices.

At some point I heard the night float, Kevin, speaking to someone outside the door of my room.

"Just wanted to make sure you saw that Mr. West is on the precautions for a resistant staph infection."

"They're not treating this infection, are they?"

"No."

"They were all so hot and bothered about getting blood cultures drawn on him. What a bunch of hypocrites."

"Well, at least we'll protect the other patients by having him on precautions. That's medicine. I'm glad I only have to do a rotation through here. I'll stay with pediatrics anytime."

"Yeah, you people take care of them through their teens and then send them to us to die."

"Hey, guys, what's up?"

"Not much, Mike. What brings you to this floor?"

"I'm looking for some gram stain in the lab. By the way, did you hear the gomer on the fifth floor died a few hours ago? I think her name was Mrs. Nelson."

"She finally went, huh?"

"You bet, Kevin. Listen, I'm in the ICU this month, and I don't want any of your vegetables up there. Send them someplace else to get watered. My new resident in the ICU says he's only going to accept viable protoplasm."

"We'll believe it when we see it. That resident will get pressured into taking admissions that you think are dirtballs."

"We'll see, but he won't admit them without a fight from me first. I'm sick and tired of taking care of gomers who just die anyway. I've got to run. Catch you fellas later."

Oh, God, I felt so angry. The way they talked about patients—about me—as if we were no longer human. What gave these young men the right to treat us as though we're just protoplasm? Is that what we become when we can't function on our own? I wished to God I could talk. I would put those bastards in their place.

Tranquil? Mary Ellen said I looked tranquil. After hearing those guys in the hall, I had such a surge of adrenaline and anger throughout me that I could almost move my fingers. But who the hell would see it anyway? People will only come in now when they have to. Now that I'm on precautions, I won't even get turned half as much.

———

"Oh, Christ, Susan, Mr. West is loaded with secretions. But it can't be helped. We got two admissions right in a row. One was the DT'er who took up practically our entire evening. And Mr. West is low on the priority list."

"I know, but it just doesn't seem right that his secretions are let go until he practically drowns in them."

"All we can do is our best, and right now, we are taking care of Mr. West. Late, but we managed to get in here. I know some nurses that would not even bother if they were running late."

"Still, I feel guilty."

"I know you do, Sue. Let's position him on his side. Maybe he won't build up the secretions so quickly."

"By the way, the supervisor came by a little while ago. She told me that there were only going to be two nurses on tonight."

"They're going to be pretty busy, and I'm sure that they will get in this room even less than we did."

"At least he'll be suctioned out good before the change of shift. Possibly, they will get back to him in the middle of the night sometime."

"I would do some overtime, but I'm not physically up for it."

"Neither am I."

A prisoner within my own flesh in a twilight sleep. I wondered when will it all end to give me the freedom I so richly deserved? I wanted so much for this all to end. Why had all this happened to me? Me, John West, a once productive human being lying helpless in bed without an ounce of ability to fight back for my life.

I wanted the end to be near. I had nothing left but my soul to heal. The healers of the sick deserted me. Do I blame them? People like me have become the ridicule of medicine.

Because of the technology we possessed, I remained on a ventilator with no functional contribution to everyday life. Medical advances and technical endeavors have created the dilemma of DNR. Question: Should we or should we not turn off the respirator? Who dares tread the still water of courage? The response was mostly: *Cover your ass.*

The first question they ask themselves is: *Are we legally responsible if we shut it off?* Who would know if you just closed the curtain around the bed? Hell, after all is said and done and there's nothing more for us, you're stuck taking care of us. We become known as gomers, protoplasm, and oh yes, I almost forgot, watered vegetables.

But what about when technical advances bring on suffering? In addition to patting themselves on the back for saving lives with their new technology, doctors should also have to acknowledge how many people they "save" continue on for days, months, or even years, dependent on that technology. I happen to be just one of the many who remained alive interminably on the ventilator, just waiting to die.

I'm luckier than most because they gave up on me in a relatively short period of time because of complications. There are some individuals who remain in intensive care units for months, being poked and prodded like pin cushions, blown up with fluid to maintain blood pressure until their skin pops, only for their eventual outcome to still be death.

Where do we draw the line? There's no one-size-fits-all. It depends on the individual situation, the state which you're in, the hospital, your family, and whether you meet the criteria for brain death.

We also become victims. One of my gripes while I was commissioner was the cost of the double-blind mechanism. It was a bill that looked good on paper, itemizing how much care went into the patient. However, in reality, much of the care itemized on a patient's bill was duplicated to increase the cost, which in turn increased the revenue credit from the insurance provider. I had investigated one such patient who was in a coma for over a year. It turned out the billing department was told to *beef up the bill a little*. I was appalled, but it was true.

Further investigation led me to City Hall, where it all originated. Orders came from there long before Bill and I took office, and there wasn't a damn thing we could do about it. It had been done for years and years. No wonder there was such chaos when we had to lay off workers in housekeeping, laundry, etc. They too were the victims of a corrupt bureaucracy.

All those memories went through my brain that night. As commissioner I hadn't fully understood that we were all players in the game of life and death and at the mercy of the omnipotent few who possess transient supremacy over the vulnerable, weak, and wounded.

I finally drifted into sleep, a respite from all these memories.

I heard Sam's voice, which sounded slightly muffled, probably from wearing a mask.

"How are things today, Johnny? We all had dinner at Mary Ellen's mother's last night. Everyone was asking about you, and they're all praying for you. It did us all good to be out for the evening, but there was a hole in our hearts without you there. It's just not the same. You're the glue. There were moments of laughter about the past, but there was also a sense of emptiness thinking about the future, which is impossible to imagine without you. I wish it were me lying in that bed instead of you. I love you so."

"Excuse me, Dr. West. I don't mean to interrupt, but housekeeping is here to wash down the walls and floors. They use a special solution that helps minimize the chance of the infection spreading."

"Sure, I understand. How long will they be?"

"No more than twenty minutes."

"Okay. I'll be back. Will you beep me when they finish?"

"Sure."

"Okay, Johnny, I'll be back soon."

I felt uneasy when Sam left, wishing he had stayed with me.

"Okay, fellas, the room is all yours. Please be very careful of the wires and machinery."

"Will do, ma'am."

"Come to the desk and let me know when you're finished, okay?"

"Sure."

The cleaning crew mostly spoke Spanish, with a little broken English here and there. Either way, I couldn't make out what they were saying. But I swore I could feel them staring at me, watching me, especially when they weren't talking.

For a while all I heard was the clanging of metal buckets and the slapping of mops going back and forth. When they started talking again, it sounded like a heated disagreement or argument. I sensed they were arguing about me, but why would that be? It went on long enough for a nurse to step into the room and ask them to keep their voices down.

"Also, your supervisor just called. He wants you both to go down to the emergency room immediately to clean one of the trauma rooms for an admission."

"Okay, Miss," one answered.

"Is it all right to visit with Mr. West now?"

It was Mary Ellen, and I felt my uneasiness lift.

"Just as soon as housekeeping is finished disinfecting. You can wait down the hall for a moment."

"Okay. Thank you."

I heard them emptying the buckets, meaning they were packing up. I wanted them to hurry so Mary Ellen could be with me. I heard footsteps walking away, and the room was silent except for the rhythmic whoosh of the ventilator. Then the sound stopped, and it became harder to breathe.

It became harder to take air in. With each exhale I could feel myself slowly suffocating. It felt as though a great weight was crushing my chest. I started to fade into a different kind of darkness, a nothingness. Then I was floating and could look down and see my lifeless body motionless on the bed, still attached to the ventilator. I also saw a man in work clothes leave the room as Mary Ellen entered.

She walked over to me, her expression changing to disbelief and then grief as she shouted my name over and over. She spotted the disconnected plug just as the nurse came running into the room. Mary Ellen pointed, and the nurse picked up the plug with a look of shock and plugged it back into the wall socket. The ventilator moaned, then began to provide its eternal breath again. But I didn't need it anymore.

I was finally, mercifully free.

Afterword

As a young nurse at a large city hospital, I would come in on the day shift and find patients who had died alone during the night. There was a nursing shortage at the time, and a petition went around describing what was going on inside the hospital with these patients. It was published as an editorial in the Boston Globe. The head nurse who started the petition was fired. I quickly learned about City Hall politics. She never got her position back even though her brother was a doctor.

With the advancement of CPR, intubation, and ventilators many patients who had suffered a cardiac arrest and were resuscitated with minimal brain activity lingered in the rooms on the floors for many months. It bothered me to hear and see how some of these patients were treated on rounds. They were once someone's mother or father who before their catastrophic event had lived a full life. Thus *DNR* was written.

I have been a registered nurse for fifty-two years. My passion was taking care of patients at the bedside where you not only made a difference but had more quality time with your patients. I was a Nurse Manager for many years in the Coronary Intensive Care unit, Electrophysiology Lab, and Progressive Care Unit in a Level 1 Trauma city hospital. I retired last year as a Director of Case Management in a designated Covid 19 Hospital and witnessed firsthand the destruction of human life the Covid protein has caused.

About the Author

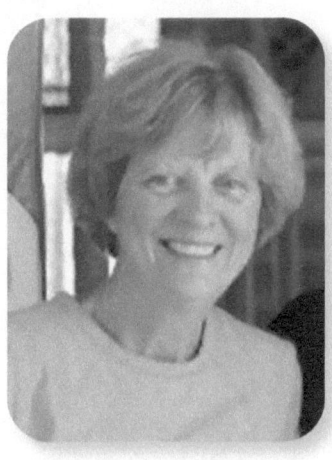

Geraldine M. McEachern was a registered nurse for more than fifty years. Her passion was bedside care of patients, where she could spend quality time and make personal connections that brought comfort to those she tended. She was a nurse manager for many years in a Coronary Intensive Care Unit, an electrophysiology lab, and a progressive care unit in a Level 1 trauma hospital. Prior to her retirement in January 2022, she was director of Case Management in a designated COVID-19 hospital.

DNR is her debut novel.

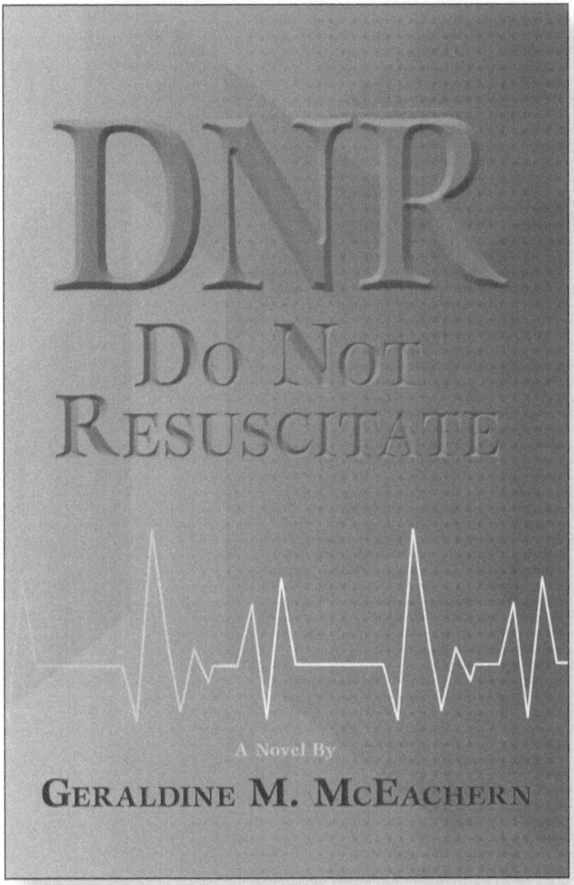

DNR, *Do Not Resuscitate*
Geraldine M. McEachern

Publisher: SDP Publishing
Also available in ebook format

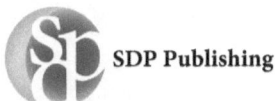
SDP Publishing

www.SDPPublishing.com
Contact us at: info@SDPPublishing.com